Lange Review:
CT Clinical Concepts and
Imaging Applications Manual with
Registry Review

Lange Review: CT Clinical Concepts and Imaging Applications Manual with Registry Review

Authors

Michael L. Grey, PhD, RT(R)(MR)(CT), FASRT
Former Professor of Radiologic Sciences
Former Program Director MRI/CT Specialization
Southern Illinois University
Carbondale, Illinois

W. Zachary Rich, JD, MBA, MS Ed., RT(R)(CT)(MR)
Attorney/Senior Conflict Analyst
MRI/CT Technologist

New York   Chicago   San Francisco   Athens   London   Madrid   Mexico City
Milan   New Delhi   Singapore   Sydney   Toronto

1 2 3 4 5 6 7 8 9   DSS   28 27 26 25 24 23

ISBN 978-1-264-63114-8
MHID 1-264-63114-6

This book was set in Minion Pro Regular by KnowledgeWorks Global Ltd.
The editors were Sydney Keen and Christie Naglieri.
The production supervisor was Rick Ruzycka.
Project management was provided by Nitesh Sharma, KnowledgeWorks Global Ltd.
The cover designer was W2 Design.
This book is printed on acid-free paper.

Library of Congress Cataloging-in-Publication Data

Names: Grey, Michael L., author. | Rich, W. Zachary, author.
Title: Lange review. CT clinical concepts and imaging applications manual
    with registry review / authors, Michael L. Grey, W. Zachary Rich.
Other titles: CT clinical concepts and imaging applications manual with
    registry
Description: New York : McGraw Hill, [2023] | Includes bibliographical
    references and index.
Identifiers: LCCN 2022027093 (print) | LCCN 2022027094 (ebook) | ISBN
    9781264631148 (paperback ; alk. paper) | ISBN 1264631146 (paperback ;
    alk. paper) | ISBN 9781264632480 (ebook)
Subjects: MESH: Tomography, X-Ray Computed—methods | Patient Care—methods
    | Examination Questions
Classification: LCC RC78.7.T6 (print) | LCC RC78.7.T6 (ebook) | NLM WN
    18.2 | DDC 616.07/5722—dc23/eng/20220727
LC record available at https://lccn.loc.gov/2022027093
LC ebook record available at https://lccn.loc.gov/2022027094

Contents

Contributing Author

Dr. Jagan Mohan Ailinani
CT and MRI Contrast Agents

Preface

The purpose in writing the *CT Clinical Concepts and Imaging Applications Manual with Registry Review* textbook is to provide a clinically oriented book for individuals entering into the medical imaging field of computed tomography. This book is designed with the learner in mind and is laid out in three main sections. The first section focuses on topics like patient care and preparation, contrast media, and medicolegal issues.

The second section addresses common imaging applications performed in CT today. Each imaging application includes concise information on indications for performing the examination, patient/part positioning, breathing instructions, scan range, gantry angulation, slice thickness, table movement, windowing, contrast media, and radiation reduction suggestions. In addition, CT images are provided to support each application.

Finally, the third section is comprised of 250 multiple-choice questions covering a wide range of topics to help the learner prepare for the American Registry of Radiologic Technologists (ARRT) examination. Of those 250 questions, 50 are image based. Finally, an answer explanation sub-section is used as an answer key and resource to better understand the correct answer.

The intent of this textbook is to be used as a supplement during either a classroom lecture or to assist the student while attending their clinical internship.

Michael L. Grey
W. Zachary Rich

Acknowledgments

In reflecting on the journey in the development of the *CT Clinical Concepts and Imaging Applications Manual with Registry Review*, I would like to say thank you to the editorial staff at McGraw-Hill, especially Ms. Sydney Keen. The many tasks involved in writing one book can be challenging, however, working on two books (*MRI Clinical Concepts and Imaging Applications Manual with Registry Review*) simultaneously is crazy insane. To those who encouraged me to finish these books, you made the journey easier – thank you!

Finally, to Zach Rich, an individual with many titles and a lot of letters behind his name. To me, he was a student, a teaching assistant, and now an author. I have seen this young man accomplish much. Thank you.

Michael – a.k.a. "the Tutelar"

I want to start off by thanking my wonderful wife, Madelaine, and my parents, Jeff and Carol. You were incredibly supportive and understanding of the countless hours it took to put together not only one textbook, but two (*MRI Clinical Concepts and Imaging Applications Manual with Registry Review* and *CT Clinical Concepts and Imaging Applications Manual with Registry Review*). I would like to also thank Jack Bryant, Judd Hill, and Anwar Hanna for their help. You were the best technologists and people I have had the pleasure of working with. Jack, I appreciate your friendship and support over the many years we worked together and also your help with this project. To my co-author, Michael Grey (a.k.a. "the Tutelar"), thank you so much for your guidance and encouragement over the years. We began this textbook project many years ago and it is such a relief to finally see it through. Thank you for pushing me to do more, both professionally and personally. Simply put, from the Tutelee to the Tutelar, thank you. I would like to also thank the publishing team. I appreciate your work taking rough drafts and molding them into amazing final manuscripts. Finally, thank you Lord for your guidance, answered prayers, and healing.

Zach

Lange Review:
CT Clinical Concepts and
Imaging Applications Manual with
Registry Review

PART I

Introduction to CT Imaging Applications

1

CT Patient Care and Preparation

INTRODUCTION

The role of the CT technologist is multifaceted and requires them to be versatile in the performance of their job. In addition to performing the specific examination ordered by the referring physician, the technologist must be sensitive to the needs of the patient. In this section, discussion topics will focus on various aspects surrounding the actual examination being performed.

FACTORS INFLUENCING EFFECTIVE COMMUNICATION

Effective communication is very important when relating to patients. When meeting and preparing the patient for their examination, realize that each person is uniquely different in how they understand, communicate, and function. The technologist should be sensitive to these differences and adjust the conversation accordingly. These differences may vary depending on many factors, such as the individual's values, development, gender, age, sociocultural background, and perceptions. To better communicate with individuals and, more specifically, to help the patient successfully complete the examination ordered and have a positive experience in an imaging facility, the technologist should consider these factors.

The values of an individual are based on the things they consider important in life. These values define their beliefs, ideals, and desires and have a major influence on their behavior and attitude. Listening to an individual and what they talk about will usually provide a sense of their values, interests, and previous experiences.

The personal development of an individual varies depending on their age, experiences, education, various abilities and disabilities, and maturity. Age alone cannot determine

maturity. Some children may be very mature for their age, whereas some young adults may appear childish in their behavior. The level of education an individual has achieved may influence their level of understanding. The technologist should choose their words wisely to improve their communication with their patients.

Gender differences between men and women may be seen in their communication style and how each hears or listens to what is being discussed. Cultural differences when working with individuals from other countries may also affect the communication process. Being knowledgeable and respectful of these differences will be greatly appreciated and benefit the outcome of the examination.

While patients come in all ages, being cognizant of whether the patient is understanding the content of the conversation is foundational to the successful experiences of the individual. Modifying communication skills to the needs and level of understanding of the patient will be much appreciated. For children and patients under the age of consent, communication needs to be flexible and also include parents or legal guardians.

The patient's values and sociocultural background are based on their general understanding and preconceptions surrounding their world and their personal experiences. Sociocultural differences may be seen in the individual's language skills, such as in their accent, the gestures they make, and the attitudes they demonstrate.

An individual's perceptions, which may be based on their physical senses, such as gut feelings, observations, or hearsay, can affect how they understand and interpret information and their surrounding environment. Trying to communicate better with individuals, accepting them as they are, and trying to better understand their concerns, fears, and previous experiences will help the patient complete the exam. The successful outcome of the examination being performed and the individual's experience rest largely on the initial care, skills, and character demonstrated by the technologist. As part of the health care team and as a health care professional, technologists should always conduct themselves in a professional manner. This includes addressing individuals with honorific titles (eg, Mr, Mrs, Ms, Dr, Sir, and Ma'am), maintaining eye contact during conversation, answering questions clearly and at a level the individual can understand, maintaining good personal hygiene, and wearing modest attire. Ideally, the way a technologist is seen in their workplace is also demonstrated in the public setting.

STYLES OF COMMUNICATION

In all basic forms of communication, there are at least 2 individuals involved, a sender and a receiver. As communication occurs, there is a message, such as an instruction, given by the sender and feedback from the receiver. Interpersonal communication is performed verbally and nonverbally. While conversing with the patient, it is important for technologists to be aware of the nonverbal actions being projected by both the patient and themselves. Points to consider in verbal communication include vocabulary, denotation and connotation, pacing, intonation, clarity, and timing. Points to consider in nonverbal communication include appearance, posture, facial expression, eye contact, body gestures, touch, sounds, and personal space (Table 1–1).

Verbal Communication

Verbal communication includes the spoken and written word. Choosing words wisely and appropriately and pronouncing them clearly at an understandable level will help to ensure good communication. In addition, the manner in which these words are spoken can also assist in the communication process. The technologist should also realize that some words can have

several meanings and be careful how these words may be interpreted to avoid any misunderstanding or confusion regarding what is said.

One example of a word that has a variety of meanings is *sports* (eg, baseball or basketball). When using the word *sports*, one person may be thinking of baseball, while another may be thinking of basketball. In a more practical example, the use of the word *okay* or the phrase "you are doing fine" may communicate the wrong message to the individual. For example, imagine how embarrassing it was for the following radiography student working alongside a technologist as the technologist was telling the patient what to do while positioning the patient for a posteroanterior upright chest exam. Several times during the instructions, the technologist said the word *okay*. After the patient was positioned for the upright chest exam, the technologist and student turned and walked back to the operator console to select the technique to use. During their walk back to the console, the technologist said the word *okay* again. As they rounded the corner to the console and looked through the window, they noticed that the patient was not at the upright chest board; instead, the patient was right behind them in the x-ray control area. Shocked and confused, the technologist asked the patient why he had followed them. The patient responded that he had heard them say "okay" and thought the exam was complete and that he was supposed to follow them out of the exam room. As a habit, the overuse of the word *okay* misled the patient to think the exam was finished because the technologist used the word *okay* to transition to performing the next step of the exam and then again before asking the patient to take a deep breath. Likewise, using the phrase "you're doing fine" with a patient may communicate the message that the patient does not need the examination or that the examination appears to be normal. A better and more specific phrase would be, for example, "You are doing a good job holding still." Miscommunication can lead the patient to question the doctor's report, especially if the report is found to be pathologically positive.

Pacing or talking too fast may inhibit the individual's ability to clearly understand or remember what is being said. It is important to speak slowly so that words are processed clearly and understood. In addition, elderly patients may not hear as well as younger patients, and others with a hearing impairment may better understand what is being said by reading lips. Reading lips may also be difficult and lead to confusion since many healthcare workers wear face masks.

The tone or intonation of the communication can also be misleading. The technologist's emotions, feelings, or fatigue may influence the way they express what they are saying to the patient. The technologist must always be aware of how they are expressing the communication and how it is being perceived by the patient. Is the patient perceiving anger, frustration, or joy? What is the technologist perceiving about the patient? Sometimes, it is helpful to empathize with the patient

TABLE 1–1 • Key Points of Verbal and Nonverbal Communication	
Verbal	**Nonverbal**
• Vocabulary	• Appearance
• Denotation and connotation	• Posture and gait
• Pacing	• Facial expression
• Intonation	• Eye contact
• Clarity	• Body gestures
• Timing	• Touch
	• Sounds
	• Personal space

and try to understand what the patient may be going through or other issues in their life. As a word of caution, an expression such as, "I know what you're dealing with" may not be ideal. For example, if the patient has been diagnosed with cancer and the technologist has never had cancer, how could the technologist possibly know what the patient is dealing with? Even if the technologist had experienced cancer, the technologist could still only understand what it felt like to be a cancer patient, but they could never fully understand the degree of pain and suffering the patient is experiencing.

The clarity of what is being communicated will help in reducing confusion. Technologists should try to choose their words and sentences so they are short and to the point. Their words should be clearly enunciated (especially for those with difficulty hearing) to improve communication.

Small adjustments by technologists in how they communicate may have a big effect on how well patients understand what is being said and will demonstrate the technologist's concern and care for them. The patient's experience will greatly affect how they view the imaging facility. If it is a good experience, the imaging facility will be highly thought of and much appreciated.

Nonverbal Communication

An individual's appearance is the first thing noticed in an interpersonal encounter. Many physical characteristics, such as clothing, grooming, and physical well-being, contribute to forming first impressions.

The posture and gait of an individual may be indications of their emotions, self-concept, and quality of health. While observing an individual's posture and gait should not be considered as the sole basis for assessing their overall health, they may provide a clue to the individual's well-being.

Facial expressions can reflect many emotions, ranging from sadness to happiness. Additional expressions that may be noticed include fear, pain, and anger. Paying attention to an individual's facial expressions may provide information that can benefit the communication process. In addition, technologists should be aware of their own facial expressions and the message they are sending to the patient or family members. What patient would want their technologist to have a sad or unhappy expression on their face? Think about what your facial expression communicates to your patient and others around you.

In addition to being an important part of facial expressions, eye contact can indicate a willingness to communicate. Establishing eye contact during a conversation demonstrates respect for and a desire to listen to the other person. Likewise, a lack of eye contact may communicate a lack of interest, lack of confidence, anxiety, or disrespect for the other person. It is important to note that eye contact may be seen differently by various cultures. The technologist should be aware of the cultural differences and act accordingly.

Body gestures, such as pointing a finger, having arms folded across the chest, hand and arm movements, tapping a leg, and rolling the eyes, may have specific meanings in the communication process. Facial expressions along with a person's posture and gait work together to create a specific message.

Touch is a more personal form of communication. In medical imaging, touching a patient is necessary in positioning the patient. Touching can send a variety of messages to the patient or family member, such as emotional support and encouragement. Holding the hand of a grieving patient can often show understanding better than words. Touching that occurs when shaking hands during a greeting or putting an arm around a patient to assist them with getting up on the patient's table for an examination is usually acceptable. Although some individuals and cultures may be unfamiliar to the technologist, it is important for the technologist to be aware of and sense the comfort level of the individual. Prior to touching a patient to help in positioning, the technologist should always ask permission and explain where they need to touch the patient and the reason. This demonstrates respect for the individual and improves the communication between the technologist and the patient. If family members, such as parents, are nearby, they will appreciate the thoughtfulness in asking permission.

In many situations, feelings and thoughts may be communicated through various types of sounds. These sounds include sighing, moaning, exhaling heavily, and crying. For example, a sigh may indicate relief or weariness. The technologist should observe all forms of nonverbal communication to facilitate better communication with individuals. Likewise, the sounds the technologist makes affect the communication with patients. Consider what the patient might feel or think if they ask a question and the technologist gives a sigh. Is it a sigh of boredom, frustration, or indifference? What will the patient think about the technologist and their facility? What if the patient fills out an evaluation form following their experiences in your care during their examination?

The space or distance between the technologist and an individual may be referred to as "personal space." If the personal space between individuals is invaded by decreasing this space, the patient may feel uncomfortable and threatened. Technologists are often used to being very close to patients when positioning them; however, patients may not be as comfortable with this proximity. Again, it is advised that the technologist always respect the patient and clearly communicate in a manner that will reduce a patient's discomfort.

In medical imaging, communicating with the patient and possibly the patient's family members, such as parents or legal guardians, is a process of social interaction where the technologist endeavors to gain the trust and cooperation of the patient. The technologist should understand that, for many people, being a patient can be a stressful experience that may not allow the patient to be seen at their best. Using verbal and nonverbal communication, the technologist begins the patient encounter by introducing themselves to the patient and explaining the examination in a step-by-step process, pausing at times to allow the patient to better understand and retain the information. Time and encouragement should also be provided for the patient to ask questions.

PHYSICAL SCREENING AND ASSESSMENT OF THE PATIENT

A thorough medical history prior to beginning any CT examination should be obtained to become more familiar with the following patient characteristics: (1) renal function; (2) presence of thyroid disease; (3) adverse reactions to contrast media; (4) oral administration of contrast media; (5) metallic objects in the area to be scanned; (6) intravenous (IV) injection site selection; and (7) blood clotting factors.

Renal Function

Because many of the CT examinations performed require an IV injection of an iodinated contrast agent and because contrast agent is filtered and excreted primarily via the urinary system, assessing the renal function of the patient is essential. Asking the patient about any known history of allergies or any past allergic reactions is a good starting point. However, some patients may not recall specific events, such as a previous allergic reaction to an IV contrast agent. As a precaution, it is important to realize that some individuals still use terms that are incorrect (eg, dye). Using terms that are not accurate can be misleading or confusing and can cause additional concern for the patient. As professionals, using the correct and current terminology shows respect for the patient while better educating them regarding the procedure that is being performed on them.

Reviewing the results of recent blood tests evaluating the patient's blood urea nitrogen, serum creatinine, and calculated estimated glomerular filtration rate (eGFR) will provide information regarding their renal function and the risk of contrast-induced acute kidney injury (CI-AKI) prior to administering the iodinated IV contrast agent. The eGFR is the more accurate of these tests in predicting the patient's true glomerular filtration rate.

Specifically, CI-AKI is used to describe a sudden deterioration in renal function that is caused by the IV administration of an iodinated contrast agent; it is a subgroup of contrast-associated acute kidney injury (CA-AKI). CA-AKI is a general term used to describe a sudden deterioration in renal function that occurs within 48 hours following the administration of an IV iodinated contrast agent.

Thyroid Disease

Patients with hyperthyroidism can develop a condition known as thyrotoxicosis (too much thyroid hormone in the body) following an IV injection of iodinated contrast agent. Hyperthyroidism is most often caused by an autoimmune condition called Graves disease.

A rare condition known as a thyroid storm or thyroid crisis can be life threatening. Patients with hyperthyroidism may be at greater risk of experiencing a thyroid storm. In these patients, the use of an iodinated contrast agent should be avoided. Blood tests (eg, T_3, T_4, and thyroid-stimulating hormone [TSH]) are used to evaluate the function of the thyroid gland.

Proper sequencing of a patient who needs multiple examinations should be considered when scheduling. As a precaution, patients scheduled to receive radioactive iodine should not undergo contrast-enhanced CT exams without prior physician approval. This may cause the diagnostic scintigraphy study to be rendered nondiagnostic for several weeks following iodinated contrast media administration. Likewise, injecting iodinated contrast media into a patient undergoing thyroid cancer treatment may seriously influence the overall treatment and prognosis of the disease.

Adverse Reactions to Contrast Media

A previous known reaction to an iodinated contrast agent is a contraindication to performing the CT examination with IV contrast. As always, the technologist should contact the radiologist to discuss any concerning patient issues. In addition, documentation of that conversation should be included in the patient's chart. Information should include the radiologist consulted, date and time of the conversation, topics discussed, and outcome of the conversation. The technologist should sign and date and time the conversation in the patient's chart. If for some reason the patient's chart is not available, the technologist should still make note of the conversation in the event there are any questions or concerns later.

Metformin (eg, Glucophage) is an oral antihyperglycemic agent used to treat patients with type 2 diabetes. For patients who are taking metformin and have been scheduled for a CT exam requiring an iodinated contrast agent and who have renal function within normal limits, metformin should be discontinued for 48 hours following the examination. Metformin may be restarted 48 hours after the exam if the patient's renal function is acceptable. A review of your imaging department's guidelines for procedures is recommended to provide further instructions and to maintain current practices.

Finally, patients with a history of asthma have an increased likelihood of experiencing an allergic type of contrast reaction. These patients may be more likely to develop bronchospasm.

Oral Administration of Contrast Media

For examinations that require an oral contrast agent, the patient will need to fast for some time prior to the scheduled exam. In addition, they may need to arrive at least an hour before their exam begins to finish drinking any additional liquid contrast media. Using the correct contrast media is very important. Contact the reading radiologist regarding any surgery, suspected bowel perforation, or fistula the patient may have.

Metallic Objects

When preparing the patient for the ordered exam, ask them to remove all metallic objects in the scan range before positioning them on the scanner table. This will help reduce image artifacts, which may result in reduced image quality.

IV Injection

Preparing to begin an IV saves time, allows for better organization, and appears more professional to the patient. Establishing a routine or having a checklist of what is needed will help facilitate this process. A point to consider is whether the contrast agent is to be hand injected or whether a power injector is going to be used. Once that decision is clarified, then select the gauge of IV catheter, 3 short (approximately 3 inches long) pieces of tape to secure the IV catheter (paper tape will secure the catheter and not hurt the patient when being removed), 2 × 2 gauze pads, and a bandage (post removal of the catheter). In addition, the type and amount of IV contrast agent will need to be determined, a saline chaser should be drawn up, and the IV tubing will need to be connected and flushed to remove all air and decrease the chance of an air embolus entering the patient. At your operator console (for power injector use), select the flow rate for the contrast agent and saline chaser.

Prior to inserting the IV, inform the patient about what you are going to be doing and what type of CT examination has been ordered, and provide a basic overview of how the examination will be performed. When informing the patient on the specific details of the examination, include information on positioning issues, breathing instructions, the importance of holding still, approximate length of examination time, where the technologist will be during the actual scan, and how to communicate with the technologist during the examination. In addition, repeat key points for the patient, ask the patient if they have any questions, and encourage them during the examination to improve the overall scanning experience for the patient.

At this point, ask the patient if they have a preference on where they would like you to start the IV. This is known as IV site selection, and usually, the antecubital area is used. The veins in this area are larger and can better tolerate the amount of contrast media injected per second (flow rate) than the veins in the back of the hand and is also less painful for the patient.

Some patients want to know what they can do to help in the examination. This is a great time to get them involved simply by saying, "Please hold still, but if you experience any pain or discomfort at the injection site, please let me know."

Blood Clotting Factors

Patients on blood thinners (anticoagulants), such as warfarin (Coumadin), heparin, or clopidogrel (Plavix), should consult their medical doctor about withholding these medications prior to any invasive procedure performed (eg, biopsy/drainage) and then restarting their blood thinner. Discussing the management of their blood thinners with their medical doctor is important and will assure a better outcome during and following their procedure.

Prior to beginning any invasive procedure, such as a biopsy or drainage, the patient's blood clotting capabilities, should be reviewed. The 2 blood tests commonly used to evaluate coagulation status are the prothrombin time (PT), which measures the integrity of the extrinsic system, and the partial thromboplastin time (PTT) or activated partial thromboplastin time (aPTT), which are used to test the integrity of the intrinsic system. The aPTT is more sensitive when monitoring patients on heparin therapy. In addition, a complete blood count (CBC) will include the patient's platelet (thrombocyte) count. A normal platelet count is between 150,000 and 400,000/μL of blood. A platelet count higher than 450,000/μL is known as thrombocytosis. A platelet count lower than 150,000/μL is called thrombocytopenia. A low platelet count may result in excessive bleeding.

The normal PT (or average time for blood to clot) is about 10 to 13 seconds. A higher PT indicates that the blood takes longer than usual to clot, whereas a lower (quicker) PT means the blood clots more quickly than normal. The average PTT ranges from 60 to 70 seconds, whereas the average aPTT ranges from 30 to 40 seconds.

Blood clotting and coagulation status values need to be approved by the radiologist prior to beginning the procedure.

Following the Examination

At the conclusion of the examination, ask the patient how they are doing. Compliment the patient regarding their participation in completing the examination and obtaining good-quality images for the doctor to review. Because they have been lying down for some time, helping them to sit up on the edge of the patient's table will be appreciated and will allow the technologist to assess the patient's stability before getting off the table.

Patients may inquire as to the results of the examination and where to go next. The technologist should be familiar with instructions that answer these types of questions. Usually, the patient is scheduled to see the ordering physician, at which time the results of the examination (ie, report) will be discussed. If the technologist sees something which may be of concern on the images during the examination that needs to be reviewed immediately by the radiologist before the patient leaves the CT suite, the technologist may ask the patient to have a seat in the waiting room until further instructions are provided.

Documenting specific information in the patient's chart regarding the examination should be performed by the technologist primarily involved with imaging the patient. This process should only focus on key components of the examination and may be as short and simple as stating the patient's tolerance of the procedure and specific details of the venipuncture procedure (eg, anatomic injection site, gauge of catheter, amount of contrast media used and flow rate, any complications encountered). Because contrast agents are drugs, they should be documented by the individual who started the IV and injected the contrast agent. Fortunately, in most cases, the patient will tolerate the injection of the contrast agent with no complications.

2
CT and MRI Contrast Agents

Technologists working in computed tomography (CT) or magnetic resonance imaging (MRI) are responsible for performing a wide variety of examinations on a diverse population of patients. Many of these examinations require the use of a contrast agent. It is very important, therefore, that the technologist has a working knowledge of how to perform venipuncture and how to safely administer the specific contrast agent required. To safely administer a contrast agent, the technologist must be able to determine 5 things:

- The specific contrast agent to be used
- The correct amount to be used
- The appropriate injection site
- The correct injection rate
- The appropriate gauge of the intravenous (IV) needle to be used

Upon the completion of the examination, all pertinent details of the venipuncture and administration of the contrast agent should be documented in the patient chart by the technologist, along with the overall patient outcome. To ensure the safety of the patient, it would be beneficial for the technologist to have an overview of the main points to consider prior to using either a CT or an MRI contrast agent.

CT CONTRAST AGENTS

Water-soluble contrast agents, which consist of molecules containing atoms of iodine, are used extensively in CT. Although the risk of adverse reaction is low, there is a real risk inherent in their use, which can run from mild to life threatening. Due to these safety risks, newer but more expensive, low-osmolar contrast agents have replaced the older, cheaper, high-osmolar ionic contrast agents. Adverse side effects are uncommon for these agents, ranging from 5% to 12% with ionic to 1% to 3% with nonionic, low-osmolality intravascular contrast agents.

Mild reactions are the most common type of reaction and usually do not require treatment. Patients experiencing any of the typical reactions should be observed for 30 minutes following the onset to ensure that the reaction does not become more severe. Common signs and symptoms of mild reactions include the following:

- Nausea and vomiting
- Urticaria and pruritis
- Sneezing
- Itchy or scratchy throat
- Feeling warm or chills
- Headache, dizziness, anxiety, and altered taste

Moderate reactions are not life threatening but commonly require treatment for symptoms. Some of these reactions may become severe if not treated. Common signs and symptoms of moderate reactions include the following:

- Diffuse urticaria or pruritis
- Diffuse erythema with stable vital signs
- Facial edema without dyspnea
- Throat tightness or hoarseness without dyspnea
- Wheezing or bronchospasm with mild or no hypoxia
- Protracted nausea or vomiting
- Isolated chest pain
- Vasovagal reaction that requires and is responsive to treatment

Patients should be monitored until symptoms resolve. Benadryl is effective for relief of symptomatic hives. β-Agonist inhalers help with bronchospasm (wheezing), and epinephrine is indicated for laryngeal spasm. Leg elevation (Trendelenburg position) is indicated for vasovagal reactions and hypotension.

Severe reactions, which are potentially life-threatening reactions, usually occur within the first 20 minutes following the intravascular injection of contrast. Severe reactions are rare but should be recognized and treated immediately. Common signs and symptoms of severe reactions include the following:

- Diffuse edema or facial edema with dyspnea
- Diffuse erythema with hypotension
- Laryngeal edema with stridor and/or hypoxia
- Anaphylactic shock (hypotension with tachycardia)
- Vasovagal reaction resistant to treatment
- Arrhythmia
- Convulsions or seizures
- Hypertensive emergency

Severe bronchospasm or severe laryngeal edema may progress to unconsciousness, seizures, hypotension, dysrhythmias, or cardiac arrest and need for immediate cardiopulmonary resuscitation.

Local side effects, such as extravasation of the contrast agent at the injection site, may cause pain, swelling, skin slough, and deeper tissue necrosis. The affected limb should be elevated. A warm compress may help with absorption of the contrast agent, whereas a cold compress is more effective in reducing pain at the injection site. With the current use of power injectors, extra care should be taken in observing the injection site during the administration phase of the contrast agent.

Although the terms *extravasation* and *infiltration* have been used interchangeably, a difference should be noted. Infiltration is the inadvertent administration of a nonvesicant fluid (eg, normal saline) into the surrounding tissues. Extravasation is the inadvertent administration of a vesicant fluid (eg, contrast agent, chemotherapy) into the surrounding tissue. A vesicant fluid can cause necrosis or tissue damage when it escapes from the vein.

Contrast-Induced Nephropathy

Contrast-induced nephropathy (CIN) is defined as acute renal failure (sudden deterioration in renal function) occurring within 48 hours of contrast injection and is a significant source of morbidity. CIN is a subgroup of postcontrast acute kidney injury. The most prominent risk factors are diabetes and chronic renal insufficiency. Adequate hydration is essential in the prevention of CIN. Patients should be encouraged to drink several liters of water or fluid 12 to 24 hours before and after intravascular administration of contrast. As a prophylactic treatment, an IV bolus of *N*-acetylcysteine (Mucovit) may also be recommended at a dose given orally (600 mg twice daily) on the day before and on the day of contrast administration. Another option is to give 500 mL of normal saline over 30 minutes prior to the exam and 500 mL of normal saline over 4 hours after the examination.

Metformin (Glucophage)

Metformin (Glucophage) is an oral antihyperglycemic agent used to treat type 2 diabetes mellitus. It may potentially cause fatal lactic acidosis. Metformin should be discontinued for 48 hours following iodinated contrast administration and reinstated only after renal function is reevaluated and found to be normal.

Patients at high risk for adverse contrast reactions should be identified and consideration given as to whether a contrast agent should be given. In cases where administrating a contrast agent may not be in the best interest of the patient, alternative imaging such as ultrasound may be helpful. Further, it may be possible for the radiologist to monitor the noncontrast CT exam to assess the images as they are acquired. If contrast is needed, the patient should be adequately hydrated. Premedication should be considered.

Risk factors for adverse reactions to contrast agents include the following:

- Previous history of adverse reactions to IV contrast
- Clear history of asthma or allergies (a history of an allergy to shellfish or iodine is not a reliable indicator of a possible contrast reaction)
- Known cardiac dysfunction including severe congestive heart failure, severe arrhythmias, unstable angina, recent myocardial infarction, or pulmonary hypertension
- Renal insufficiency, especially in patients with diabetes mellitus
- Sickle cell disease
- Multiple myeloma
- Age over 65

All patients who receive CT contrast should be screened appropriately. For patients at risk for reduced renal function, serum creatinine and estimated glomerular filtration rate (GFR) should be obtained. Technologists need the patient's age, gender, weight, and serum creatinine to use the GFR calculator (which can be found online). Patients who have a GFR of less than 30 mL/min should not be given contrast.

Premedication has been proven to decrease but not eliminate the frequency of contrast reactions. Two regimens listed by the American College of Radiology include either (1) prednisone 50 mg taken orally at 13 hours, 7 hours, and 1 hour before contrast administration or (2) methylprednisolone 32 mg taken orally at 12 hours and 2 hours prior to contrast administration. Benadryl 50 mg orally, intramuscularly, or IV should be administered 1 hour prior to contrast for either of the regimens. In addition, nonionic low-osmolality contrast should be used with either regimen.

MRI CONTRAST AGENTS

Gadolinium chelates are the most commonly used magnetic resonance (MR) contrast agents. These agents differ based on being either ionic or nonionic and based on their osmolality and viscosity. Their distribution and elimination are very similar to water-soluble, iodine-based contrast agents used in CT. Injected IV, gadolinium chelates diffuse rapidly into extracellular fluid and blood pool spaces and are excreted by glomerular filtration. About 80% of an injected dose is excreted within 3 hours. MRI is usually done immediately after injection.

Adverse reactions to gadolinium contrast agents are quite uncommon. Common signs and symptoms of mild reactions include the following:

- Nausea and vomiting
- Headache
- Warmth or coldness at the injection site
- Paresthesia
- Dizziness
- Itching

Life-threatening reactions are rare. Gadolinium has no nephron toxicity at doses used for MRI. Because gadolinium agents are radiopaque, they have been used in conventional angiography in patients with renal impairment or severe reaction to iodinated contrast.

Nephrogenic Systemic Fibrosis

Nephrogenic systemic fibrosis, originally described in 2000, is a systemic disorder characterized by widespread tissue fibrosis following the administration of a gadolinium-based contrast agent in individuals with noticeable advanced renal failure. This disease causes fibrosis of the skin and connective tissues throughout the body. Patients affected develop skin thickening that may prevent bending and extending of joints, resulting in their decreased mobility. Affected patients also experience fibrosis that has spread to other parts of the body, such as the diaphragm, muscles of the thigh and lower abdomen, and interior areas of the lung vessels. The clinical course is progressive and fatal.

Patients at high risk for reduced renal function include those with the following risk factors:

- Age 65 or over
- Diabetes mellitus
- History of renal disease or renal transplants
- History of liver transplantation or hepatorenal syndrome

As a safety precaution, serum creatinine and estimated GFR should be obtained in all patients with reduced renal function. Patients who have a GFR of less than 30 mL/min should not be given contrast.

IV Contrast and the Pregnant Patient

The safety of fetal exposure to CT and MR contrast agents is not well described in the literature. The current recommendation is to avoid routine administration of contrast agents in pregnant patients unless the information is critical to the management of the patient (risk vs benefit). Alternate imaging studies such as ultrasound must also be considered.

3

Overview of Medical-Legal Issues in Computed Tomography for Technologists

The frequency of medical-legal issues continues to increase, including in the area of medical imaging. This chapter aims to better prepare medical imaging students and entry-level employees for the workforce and to help employers avoid ligation. The legal cases in this chapter are only examples of legal principles. It is important to note that health law is constantly changing and evolving over time. This chapter is not a substitute for legal advice.

RADIOLOGIC TECHNOLOGIST MALPRACTICE PAYMENTS

The National Practitioner Data Bank (NPDB) was established by the Health Care Quality Improvement Act of 1986.[1] The NPDB lists "adverse hospital privileging actions, professional society reports, and malpractice payments made on behalf of licensed health care practitioners."[2] Any entity, insurance company, or organization making a payment on behalf of a health care practitioner due to a malpractice settlement or judgment is required to report the payment to the NPDB.[3]

Between 1991 and 2008, a total of 155 radiologic technologist malpractice cases were reported to the NPDB.[4] Nationally, malpractice payments ranged from 2 to 16 per year.[5] Of the 155 radiologic technologist malpractice cases, 135 provided litigation information.[6] Ninety-four percent of the 135 cases (ie, 127 cases) resulted in negotiated settlements, and the remaining 6% (ie, 8 cases) resulted in court judgments.[7] Eighty-eight percent (ie, 137 cases) were paid by insurance companies or insurance guarantee funds, 8% (ie, 13 cases) were paid by self-insurance, and 3% (ie, 5 cases) were paid by state medical malpractice funds.[8]

Radiologic technologist malpractice payments ranged from $750 to $11.5 million, with a median payment of $57,500 and only 2 payments exceeding $1 million.[9] Extracting the 2 outlier payments of over $1 million, the mean payment was $177,598.[10] By comparison, during the same period, 325,104 malpractice cases were recorded in the NPDB for all health care providers, with a range of $50 to $27.5 million.[11] It is difficult to explain the infrequency of medical malpractice cases against radiologic technologists, especially because the number of technologists and the nation's population have increased between 1991 and 2008.[12]

The most probable cause for the stability and frequency in medical malpractice cases against radiologic technologists may be the "shielding technologists receive from the hospitals and physicians with whom they are affiliated."[13] The injured plaintiff will often look to other codefendants for the capital to meet a settlement or jury verdict, even though the technologist was the party against whom negligent conduct was alleged.[14] Hospitals and radiologists take on a large amount of vicarious liability for the actions of technologists.[15]

A technologist is typically an "employee of a hospital, outpatient imaging facility, or radiology group."[16] Therefore, in these cases, the technologist's employer is named as a codefendant or sole defendant, rather than the technologist himself or herself.[17] The employer "becomes the deep pocket for the monies assessed by a jury or agreed on in a settlement."[18] Plaintiff's attorneys often formulate an allegation of wrongdoing to make the employer the sole or primary defendant because the technologist is less likely to have adequate assets or liability insurance to compensate the patient.[19]

Radiologists or supervising physicians are often included as codefendants or sole defendants.[20] Plaintiff's attorneys draw the physicians into the lawsuit under the legal theory of the borrowed servant doctrine, where the technologist is the "borrowed servant of the supervising physician."[21] For example, a supervising radiologist may be negligent for interpreting inadequate images acquired by a technologist.[22]

QUICK REFERENCE GUIDE TO AVOID LEGAL ISSUES

The reference guide below is a summary of the concepts that will be discussed in detail throughout this chapter and should help you avoid legal issues. If you have any questions, please review the relevant sections of this chapter. The list below is not exhaustive. After reading this chapter and spending time in the workplace, you may think of additional items to add to this list.

- Introduce yourself (name and position).
- Confirm that you have the correct patient, order, and imaging protocol.
- Explain the exam and answer the patient's questions. If you do not know the answer to a question, look it up and ask a colleague. Use correct terminology (eg, contrast media, not dye).
- Obtain patient consent to proceed with the exam. If informed consent is required, verify that it has been obtained by a physician.
- If the exam requires contrast and the patient is female, a negative pregnancy test or a refusal of pregnancy testing waiver is required. Follow the policy at your facility.
- Position the patient correctly.
- Immobilize the patient with straps, sandbags, and sponges, but be sure the patient is comfortable.
- Explain that you will need to touch the patient and explain why. Be respectful of the patient and respect their wishes. Do not just begin touching the patient without an explanation and consent.
- If the patient refuses to continue with the exam at any point, bring the patient out of the bore of the scanner and talk to the patient. Often, the patient just needs a short break and may decide to continue. If the patient refuses to continue, end the exam (within reason).
- When starting an intravenous (IV) line, explain what you are doing. Do not start an IV without notifying the patient. If a patient refuses the IV, talk to the patient. Often, the patient just needs an explanation. If the patient continues to refuse, document this in the patient's chart and follow the protocol at your facility. Often, the radiologist and/or requesting physician may wish to be notified.
- Use the correct contrast media and the correct dosage.

- Document the following in the patient's chart:
  - Document pertinent exam details.
  - Document whether contrast media was administered and information about the IV.
  - Document using correct terminology (eg, contrast media, not dye; computed tomography [CT], not computerized axial tomography [CAT] scan).
- Do not make disparaging comments about the patient to anyone.
- When using social media, refrain from posting anything about the patient or exam.

AMERICAN SOCIETY OF RADIOLOGIC TECHNOLOGISTS PRACTICE STANDARDS

The American Society of Radiologic Technologists (ASRT), the premier professional association for medical imaging technologists, has established practice standards to serve as a guide for appropriate practice.[23] These practice standards are created by the profession to govern the quality of practice, education, and service provided by those in the medical imaging profession as technologists.[24] The practice standards may be utilized by facilities to create practice parameters or as an "overview of the role and responsibilities of the individual as defined by the profession."[25] The ASRT requires that a technologist be "educationally prepared and clinically competent as a prerequisite to professional practice."[26] The practice standards may be superseded by state and federal laws, lawful institutional policies and procedures, and governmental accreditation standards.[27] It is important for technologists to understand the practice standards and keep current. Adhering to the practice standards reduces the potential for litigation and helps the technologist provide excellent patient care. The practice standards will be used throughout this chapter.

THE US LEGAL SYSTEM

The US Constitution (federal) and state constitutions divide power among the legislative, executive, and judicial branches. The federal legislative branch makes or enacts laws and has authority to confirm or reject presidential appointments and declare war. This branch includes Congress, which is divided into the Senate and House of Representatives. The federal executive branch carries out and enforces laws. This branch includes the president, vice president, cabinet, executive departments, independent agencies, and other committees and commissions. The federal judicial branch evaluates and applies laws; in other words, the judicial branch interprets and applies laws to individual cases. It also decides if laws violate the Constitution. This branch includes the Supreme Court and other federal courts. Each state has its own state constitution that is similar, if not identical, in structure to the US Constitution (ie, 3 branches of government). In addition, the specific duties of each branch (ie, legislative, executive, and judicial) of state government are similar to those of the federal government but pertain only to the state and not the federal government. For example, a state senate does not have authority to confirm or reject nominees to the US Supreme Court made by the president of the United States.

Federal law consists of the Constitution, statutes, regulations, treaties, and common law. State law consists of the state constitution, statutes, regulations, and common law. The federal government and all states, except Louisiana (which practices civil law), practice common law. The American common law system dates back to England. Common law is derived from court decisions and allows the law to adapt and grow as courts make rulings. Tort law is a function of common law that may have statutory restrictions, and it is largely a creature of state common law.

Judicial proceedings may be categorized as either civil or criminal actions. Civil actions are brought to enforce, compensate, or protect a civil right. Civil actions involve noncriminal matters, including torts (or civil wrongs). In contrast, a criminal action is brought by the government against a party so the defendant may be punished for offenses made against the public. This chapter will focus on civil actions. In a civil suit, the plaintiff is the party that brings a lawsuit in a court of law against an opposing party, the defendant. The defendant is the party being sued.

Multiple people may be joined in a lawsuit (uniting parties or claims into a single lawsuit). For example, the defendants in a radiology department lawsuit could include the hospital, radiologist, and technologist. Conversely, if multiple people were harmed by the same physician, then their lawsuits could be joined into one suit, where multiple persons would be plaintiffs. Litigation is the process of bringing a lawsuit. A lawsuit, also known as a suit, is any legal action by a party against another party in a court of law.

THEORIES OF LIABILITY

This section focuses on several important theories of legal liability that apply to technologists. Generally, liability refers to a legal responsibility, obligation, or accountability to another person. The doctrine of professional liability is important for technologists to understand. Professional liability is accountability for an injured party, so that the injured person may seek damages. Technologists are accountable to patients, physicians, and all other health care professionals and may be liable for their misconduct. Technologists should understand the following doctrines and terminology and consult employer policies regarding specific procedures and protocols.

Agency

Agency is a fiduciary relationship, which means that one party—the agent—acts on behalf of another party—the principal. In this capacity, the agent's actions or words are binding upon the principal. For example, a supervising party is held vicariously (ie, indirectly) liable for the conduct of a subordinate or associate. In other words, a hospital may be held responsible for the actions of its employees, including technologists.

Respondeat Superior

Respondeat superior (ri-**spond**-dee-at soo-**peer**-ee-ər) is a Latin phrase that means "let the superior make answer." The doctrine of respondeat superior holds an employer (ie, the principal) liable for an employee's (ie, agent's) wrongful acts, when committed in the scope of employment. The elements of a cause of action for hospital liability under respondeat superior are as follows:

1. An *employment relationship* existed between the defendant, as employer, and the employee whose negligence caused the plaintiff's injury.
2. The defendant employee was *acting within the scope of his or her employment* when they negligently caused the plaintiff's injury.
3. There is proof of all of the elements necessary to establish the employee's liability as a defendant in a negligence action.[28]

Additionally, the plaintiff will most likely want to add the employer (eg, hospital, medical center, imaging facility) to a lawsuit because the employer has deeper pockets to pay damages. Insurance companies representing hospitals or imaging facilities are poised to pay large sums of money on behalf of the defendant. It is important to think about the job security of a technologist found to be at fault, even if the lawsuit bypasses the employee and focuses on the employer. The employee could be looking for a new job, which may be difficult because the former employer would probably not give a favorable employee recommendation.

Borrowed Servant

The doctrine of borrowed servant uses the doctrine of respondeat superior to hold employers (ie, the principals) liable for the negligence of their employees (ie, agents). For example, a patient is injured because of the negligence of a CT technologist. The patient brings a lawsuit against the technologist (ie, employee) and hospital (ie, employer). Often, the charge against the employer is negligent hiring practices or negligent supervision. Physicians may also be held liable for the negligence of employees under their control.

Temporary agency is common in health care, and the lines of who is in charge may be blurry. Technologists should be mindful of who is in charge during an exam and whose orders they are following. Technologists are generally under the direction and guidance of a radiologist; however, this is often disputed. Radiologists are typically not in the control room when the exam is performed but may be liable for the negligence of a technologist. Depending on the situation, technologists may be under the direction and guidance of other physicians, such as an anesthesiologist or emergency department physician.

MEDICAL-LEGAL ISSUES

The following subsections dive deeper into the Theories of Liability and discuss medical malpractice, intentional torts, defenses to the intentional torts, res ipsa loquitor, dam ages, defenses to negligence, agency, and ethics.

Medical Malpractice

Negligence is the failure of someone to practice to the standard of care that a reasonable, minimally competent professional in that field would have provided in the same or similar circumstances. The reasonable, minimally competent professional is a hypothetical person who practices with a level of knowledge, intelligence, attention, and judgment that society requires.

Medical malpractice is a specific kind of negligence claim, also known as professional negligence. Medical malpractice is the failure of a member of the medical profession to perform a duty of skill, care, and diligence exercised by members of the same profession. The elements of medical malpractice are the same as negligence (ie, duty, breach, causation, and damages), but the conduct occurs within a professional relationship and involves questions of medical judgment. However, some state legislatures have special rules in medical malpractice cases, such as limits on damages. The following 5 elements are required to satisfy a claim of medical malpractice:

1. Professional relationship (in this case, between the technologist and patient)
2. A duty of care to the patient
3. A breach of the duty of care
4. Causation
5. Damages

All of the elements must be met and are discussed further below.

Professional Relationship

Negligence and medical malpractice are similar but have several differences. Medical malpractice claims occur "within the course of a professional relationship" and "raise questions involving medical judgment."[29] Courts ask 2 questions when assessing whether a claim is ordinary negligence or medical malpractice: (1) whether the claim occurred within the course of a professional relationship and (2) whether the claim raises questions of medical judgment beyond common knowledge and experience.[30] If the answers to both questions are yes, then the

action is considered within the realm of medical malpractice; if not, then it is ordinary negligence.[31] A professional relationship encompasses licensed health care professionals, licensed health care facilities, and agents or employees of licensed health care facilities, who owe a contractual duty to provide professional health care services.[32]

The following case example will help in differentiating between medical malpractice and negligence.[33] A plaintiff (ie, a patient) filed suit against a medical center for injuries sustained during an MRI exam. The patient was involved in an all-terrain vehicle accident and sustained an injury to her knee. The patient underwent successful surgery, and her leg was placed in a full brace. Ten days later, the patient underwent an MRI exam on the same leg. The technologists inspected, tested, and approved the leg brace to proceed with the MRI exam. As the exam began, the leg brace became attracted to the MRI unit and stuck to the bore of the unit. Movement of the leg brace caused the patient to suffer additional injuries.

The patient (ie, the plaintiff) filed suit against the medical center for ordinary negligence and breach of contract. The plaintiff argued that it was common knowledge of the general public that metallic objects, which are subject to magnetism, are not to be placed near or in the vicinity of an MRI unit. The plaintiff filed a second suit alleging medical malpractice, in conjunction with the ordinary negligence and breach of contract claims. Plaintiff argued that the defendant is liable for medical malpractice because the defendants failed to "conform and adhere to the recognized standard of acceptable professional practice and failed to give proper medical treatment to the plaintiff." The lawsuits were consolidated, and the defendant moved to have the suit dismissed. The trial court dismissed the plaintiff's claim because it did not comply with state law.

On appeal, the issue became whether the plaintiff's claims constituted ordinary negligence, medical malpractice, or both. The court determined that the distinction between ordinary negligence and medical malpractice depends on whether the acts or omissions in the complaint "involve a matter of medical science or art requiring specialized skills not ordinarily possessed by lay persons" or whether the acts or omissions may be "assessed on the basis of common everyday experience."

The court determined that the MRI technologist's evaluation of the patient prior to entering the MRI unit "required specialized expertise substantially related to the rendition of medical treatment." The technologist made a judgment regarding the amount and type of metal. These judgments are not matters that may be assessed on the "basis of common everyday experience" and require specialized training. Patient evaluation and preparation for the exam was a "substantial relationship to the rendition of medical treatment by a medical professional" and constitutes medical malpractice if it deviates from the standard of care.

The key takeaway from this example is that technologists may be liable for medical malpractice because technologists have a professional relationship with the patient and utilize special expertise when evaluating and preparing patients for exams. Although this example is from MRI, the key takeaways also apply to CT imaging. Consider the special expertise you use when evaluating and preparing patients for CT exams.

Duty of Care

The next element of malpractice (ie, professional negligence) is duty of care, which is the legal responsibility one has toward the well-being of another. The duty of care is a legal obligation set to the level of the standard of care in professional situations. The standard of care may be divided into 4 parts: (1) care in the sense of attention, caution, alertness, and diligence; (2) care through education, training, skill, or experience; (3) sound professional judgment; and (4) use of personal superior abilities.[34] Sometimes, the standard of care varies by location and region, and courts may consider staffing, resources, and training opportunities, for example; however, this does not extend to professional judgments. The standard of care is established through expert testimony.

Author Daniel Penofsky published an article entitled "Diagnostic Radiology Malpractice Litigation," in which he analyzed diagnostic radiology litigation. The article includes a list of the duties of a technologist. Generally, technologists will most likely meet the standard of care if they satisfy the typical duties of a technologist. For example, the following are specific duties of care owed by a technologist to a patient:

- Duty to test radiologic imaging equipment before its use to make certain it is functioning properly
- Duty to document the proper functioning of radiologic imaging equipment
- Duty to initiate the repair of radiologic imaging equipment found to be defective or not functioning properly
- Duty to document the repair of defective radiologic equipment
- Duty to correlate the primary or referring physician's radiologic imaging order or requisition slip with the patient to ensure that the proper patient is about to undergo the radiologic imaging study
- Duty to inquire whether the patient has suffered any allergic reactions to contrast agents or media
- Duty to follow the primary or referring physician's orders or instructions pertaining to the radiologic imaging studies to be performed
- Duty to adhere to the hospital's or private facility's policies and procedures manual or similarly titled directives governing the use and operation of radiologic equipment
- Duty to comply with applicable state and federal requirements governing the use and operation of radiologic equipment
- Duty to exercise due care, skill, and diligence in the positioning of the patient, aiming and focusing the radiologic

camera, taking diagnostic images, and taking all necessary steps and precautions to obtain radiologic films that are readable and capable of interpretation by the radiologist

- Duty to exercise due care, skill, and diligence so as not to injure the patient during the performance of the radiologic imaging study
- Duty to timely transmit the radiologic films of the correct patient to the radiologist for interpretation[35]

Although this list is not exhaustive, these duties are applicable to all technologists, no matter the modality. The duties closely align with the ASRT practice standards (see the ASRT Practice Standards for Medical Imaging and Radiation Therapy at https://www.asrt.org/main/standards-and-regulations/professional-practice/practice-standards-online). Following these duties will protect the patient and technologist and also may avoid legal issues.

Breach of Duty

The next element of professional negligence is a breach of duty. The defendant breaches their duty when, under the circumstances, their conduct falls short of the standard of care owed to the plaintiff. In other words, a breach of duty is a violation of the duty of care technologists owe to patients, physicians, and all other health care workers. The standard of care asks, "What would a reasonable health care professional, who is minimally competent and reasonably situated, do in a similar circumstance? The plaintiff (ie, the patient) must use the testimony from an expert witness to establish the standard of care and the defendant's failure to meet that standard. Generally, expert witnesses are individuals who have the required education and experiences to testify as to the subject of the lawsuit.

Causation

The next element of malpractice (ie, professional negligence) is causation. Causation is shown by evidence that the injury to the plaintiff is a natural and probable consequence of the defendant's negligence. Causation is established by showing (1) a causal connection between the defendant's breach of the duty and the resulting injury[36] and (2) that it is fair to hold the defendant responsible for plaintiff's injuries under the law.[37]

Damages

The final element of professional negligence is damages, which is the term for the monetary award after winning a lawsuit. Damages are awarded only if a physical or emotional injury is proven and was caused by the defendant's breach of duty. Damages that the plaintiff suffered must be a direct result of the injury. In tort cases, including negligence, the purpose of damages is to restore the plaintiff (ie, the patient) to status quo ante (Latin for "the way things were before"). In other words, the monetary award is to restore the plaintiff to the way he or she was before the injury. The plaintiff is potentially eligible for 2 forms of monetary damages: compensatory and punitive.

Compensatory Damages Compensatory damages are awarded to compensate the plaintiff for the harm they suffered. In personal injury cases, compensatory damages are based on economic and noneconomic losses. The plaintiff is compensated for economic losses, such as past and future medical expenses, permanent disability and disfigurement, and loss of earning capacity or reduced earning capacity. The plaintiff may also be compensated for past and future pain and suffering and loss of enjoyment.

Punitive Damages In addition to compensatory damages, punitive damages are awarded to the plaintiff and aimed at punishing the defendant for willfully or recklessly causing the plaintiff harm. The policy behind punitive damages is to penalize the defendant or to make them an example. It is intended to deter undesirable conduct. Punitive damages are only awarded in extreme cases.

Res Ipsa Loquitor: A Presumption of Negligence Based on the Injury

Res ipsa loquitor (rays **ip**-sə **loh**-kwə-tər) is a Latin phrase that means "the thing speaks for itself." Under this doctrine, the fact that an accident occurred raises enough of an inference of negligence to establish a case. It occurs when (1) an accident would not normally occur unless the defendant's (ie, hospital's) conduct was negligent; (2) the accident was caused by an agent or instrumentality under the exclusive control of the defendant; and (3) the accident was not attributable to the plaintiff (ie, the patient).[38]

The first use of the res ipsa loquitur doctrine was in *Byrne v. Boadle*.[39] In this case, the plaintiff was passing by the defendant's warehouse. A barrel of flour rolled from the defendant's shop window, fell on the plaintiff's head, and injured him. At trial, the plaintiff did not show how the barrel of flour fell from the window. The trial judge sided with the plaintiff. On appeal, the judge stated: "There are certain cases of which it may be said *res ipsa loquitur* and this seems one of them. In some cases, the Court has held that the mere fact of the accident having occurred is evidence of negligence."[40] Two years later, in the case *Scott v. London & St. Katherine Docs Co.*, Chief Justice Erle offered the first clear statement of the res ipsa loquitur doctrine:

> There must be reasonable evidence of negligence. But where the thing is shown to be under the management of the defendant or his servants, and the accident is such as in the ordinary course of things does not happen if those who have the management use proper care, it affords reasonable evidence, in the absence of explanation by the defendant that the accident arose from want of care.[41]

Res ipsa loquitur has been applied in negligence and malpractice actions.[42] Res ipsa allows plaintiffs without evidence of the elements of negligence to present their case on a suggestion of negligence. The plaintiff shows the facts and circumstances regarding the injury and makes the argument that the defendant's negligence is the reasonable cause. "It is not enough that plaintiff's counsel can suggest a possibility of negligence."[43]

The case of *Ybarra v. Spangard* is a good example of the res ipsa loquitur doctrine as applied to the medical arena.[44] In the case, plaintiff brought an action for damages for personal injuries alleged to have been caused by defendants (Dr Spangard and others) during a surgical operation.[45] Plaintiff consulted defendant Dr Tilley, who diagnosed his ailment as appendicitis, and made arrangements for an appendectomy to be performed by defendant Dr Spangard at a hospital owned and managed by defendant Dr Swift. Plaintiff entered the hospital, was given a hypodermic injection, slept, and later was awakened by Drs Tilley and Spangard and wheeled into the operating room by a nurse whom he believed to be defendant Gisler, an employee of Dr Swift. Defendant Dr Reser, the anesthetist, also an employee of Dr Swift, adjusted plaintiff for the operation, pulling his body to the head of the operating table and, according to plaintiff's testimony, laying him back against 2 hard objects at the top of his shoulders, about an inch below his neck. Dr Reser then administered the anesthetic, and plaintiff lost consciousness. When he awoke early the following morning, he was in his hospital room attended by defendant Thompson, the special nurse, and another nurse who was not made a defendant.

Plaintiff testified that, prior to the operation, he had never had any pain in, or injury to, his right arm or shoulder, but that when he awakened, he felt a sharp pain about halfway between the neck and the point of the right shoulder. He complained to the nurse and then to Dr Tilley, who gave him diathermy treatments while he remained in the hospital. The pain did not cease but spread down to the lower part of his arm, and after his release from the hospital, the condition grew worse. He was unable to rotate or lift his arm and developed paralysis and atrophy of the muscles around the shoulder. He received further treatments from Dr Tilley until March of 1940 and then returned to work, wearing his arm in a splint on the advice of Dr Spangard.

Plaintiff also consulted Dr Wilfred Sterling Clark, who had x-rays taken that showed an area of diminished sensation below the shoulder and atrophy and wasting of the muscles around the shoulder. In the opinion of Dr Clark. Plaintiff's condition was due to trauma or injury by pressure or strain applied between his right shoulder and neck. Plaintiff was also examined by Dr Fernando Garduno, who expressed the opinion that plaintiff's injury was a paralysis of traumatic origin, not arising from pathologic causes, and not systemic, and that the injury resulted in atrophy, loss of use, and restriction of motion of the right arm and shoulder.

The Supreme Court of California found for the plaintiff. The court found that every defendant in whose custody the plaintiff was placed for any period was bound to exercise ordinary care to see that no unnecessary harm came to him and each would be liable for failure in this regard. Any defendant who negligently injured him, and any defendant charged with his care who so neglected him as to allow injury to occur, would be liable. The defendant employers would be liable for the neglect of their employees, and the doctor in charge of the operation would be liable for the negligence of those who became his temporary servants for the purpose of assisting in the operation.

Defenses to Medical Malpractice and Negligence

Comparative Negligence

Comparative negligence is when the plaintiff's (ie, the patient's) own negligence comparably reduces recoverable damages. The negligence of the plaintiff is compared to the negligence of the defendant. The reduction in damages is comparable to the plaintiff's level of fault in causing the injury. Most states have adopted a form of the comparative negligence doctrine.[46] Some states only allow recovery of damages if the plaintiff's negligence is less than 50% or 51%.

For example, a patient (ie, the plaintiff) fails to disclose their full medical history to the technologist and suffers an injury as a result. The technologist may claim that the patient was comparatively negligent by not disclosing their full medical history. The court may reduce the amount the plaintiff recovers by the level of fault. Alternatively, the court could find the patient was 60% negligent because their own negligence was a part in causing the injury, and in some states, the patient may not be able to recover damages.

Assumption of the Risk

Assumption of the risk is the principle that some activities have inherent risks. A plaintiff assumes the risk and is unable to recover for the negligent conduct that causes the harm. In other words, a plaintiff may be barred from recovering damages due to an injury because they knew the risk involved. Many states have incorporated assumption of risk into comparative and contributory (see endnote) negligence.

Informed Consent

Certain exams and procedures require the patient's informed consent prior to a CT exam. The technologist must know which exams require informed consent. A majority of states have adopted the professional disclosure standard, where the duty to inform the patient is by the standard of what a reasonable medical practitioner similarly situated would disclose to the patient.[47] Testimony by an expert witness is required to establish what information should be disclosed to the patient.[48] A minority of states use a reasonable patient standard, where the standard is what a reasonable patient in the same or similar circumstance would like to know when deciding whether to undergo a proposed medical action (eg, therapy, surgery).

Informed consent must be obtained by a physician and requires the physician to discuss (1) the nature of the treatment, (2) risks and benefits of the treatment, and (3) alternative procedures and associated risks.[49] The patient must have the appropriate mental capacity to make the decision voluntarily and without coercion.[50] Many cases of battery involve physicians who perform treatments that exceed the informed consent they gave, where the patient did not consent to the new treatment.[51]

Physicians obtain informed consent because it involves the practice of medicine, and only physicians are licensed to practice medicine. The ASRT practice standards require technologists to verify informed consent has been obtained.[52] Policies and procedures for obtaining informed consent may differ among imaging facilities, but a radiologist will most likely obtain informed consent. Informed consent must be reduced to writing, and technologists must have this documentation. Performing additional unconsented procedures makes the technologist liable if something goes wrong. It is important to note that the practice standards require technologists to educate and inform the patient regarding the exam; however, only physicians are qualified to discuss treatment risks, benefits, and alternative procedures. Further, it is important for the technologist to read their employer's policies regarding informed consent.

Statutes of Limitations and Repose

Statutes of limitation and repose establish a time limit on when a plaintiff (ie, the patient) may bring a suit against a defendant. The statutes allow a plaintiff a reasonable amount of time to bring a suit. Without the time limit, a defendant could face the threat of litigation for an indefinite period of time.

Malpractice Examples

Example 1[53]

Plaintiff (ie, a patient) presented to defendant's MRI facility for imaging. Following the MRI, plaintiff, who was lying on a table, attempted to stand. Plaintiff became lightheaded, lost his balance, and fell. Plaintiff alleged that defendant's employee failed to properly assist plaintiff in standing, in violation of the duty of care. Defendant (ie, employer) contended that its technologist was making his way toward plaintiff to assist plaintiff in standing when the accident occurred and that plaintiff failed to exercise due care for his own safety by getting up too fast from a prone (lying flat and face down) position. Per plaintiff's counsel, the fact that plaintiff had preexisting back problems and that there was no permanency to plaintiff's injuries had an impact on the outcome. The jury awarded plaintiff damages.

The important takeaways from this case are that technologists need to guard against patient falls and should follow the policies and procedures of their employer. The ASRT practice standards allow the technologist to immobilize the patient for the exam. Straps and sandbags will restrict patient movement and could prevent a patient from falling off the scanner table.

Example 2[54]

Plaintiff went to defendant's MRI and CT center for an MRI examination of his lumbar spine. While being introduced into the MRI, he felt a pressure on his head and the machine continued to move, bending his head forward and to the left and injuring his neck. Plaintiff alleged that the MRI technologist did not stop when plaintiff first indicated that he was in trouble and that he was improperly positioned in the unit. Defendants contended that plaintiff's description of the occurrence was not possible, that plaintiff simply raised his head and bumped it slightly against the side of the unit, and that plaintiff did not complain of any injuries at the time of the incident. Defendants also contended that plaintiff had contacted the manager of the facility within 2 or 3 days and had only complained about being treated rudely and that he had not alleged that he had twisted his neck in the unit or alleged any problems with his neck. Defendants further contended that plaintiff had a preexisting condition, that the bump that plaintiff incurred had, at most, aggravated his condition for a short time, and that plaintiff's condition was caused by degenerative changes.

At trial, plaintiff introduced evidence to prove that the incident could have occurred as plaintiff stated and that defendant's account of what occurred was inconsistent with their actions subsequent to the incident, including the calling of a technologist to look at the unit, and plaintiff provided the testimony of an independent doctor who stated that she had contacted the facility to question them about plaintiff's incident and had informed them of the details of that incident. The case was one of credibility, and the jury evidently accepted plaintiff's statement of what had occurred even though plaintiff stated that he did not know what he had hit and could not explain how it had happened. The jury awarded plaintiff $25,000 in damages and $7000 for costs.

An important takeaway from this case is that the ASRT practice standards require technologists to provide optimal patient care and to assume responsibility for patient needs during exams. Further, technologists need to explain each step of the exam and obtain patient cooperation. When positioning the patient, it is important to respect patient comfort. A comfortable and content patient will provide for a quality exam. Remember, patients may retract consent at any time, and the technologist must respect the wishes of the patient or legal guardian.

Example 3[55]

Plaintiff sustained a right hip fracture that required surgical repair when she fell off a radiography table after undergoing a radiology exam under the care of defendants. The plaintiff claimed the defendants were vicariously liable for the radiology technologist's violation of the standard of care. She claimed the technologist failed to assist her off the radiography table. Plaintiff was legally blind. The defendants denied liability and denied that the technologist violated the standard of care. Defendants claimed that the technologist instructed the plaintiff to stay on the table until she could assist her. The jury determined that the plaintiff and the defendants were comparatively negligent (see below) and allocated 40% of the negligence to the defendants and 60% to the plaintiff. The plaintiff was awarded $72,000.

An important takeaway from this case, as stated in Example 1, is that technologists need to guard against patient falls. Technologists should follow the policies and procedures of their employer. The ASRT practice standards allow the technologist to immobilize the patient for the exam. Straps and sandbags will restrict patient movement and could prevent a patient from falling off the scanner table.

Negligent Infliction of Emotional Distress

Negligent infliction of emotional distress is another specific form of negligence and occurs when the plaintiff suffers severe emotional distress resulting from the defendant's negligence. Most courts will allow the recovery of damages when physical contact occurs or if the plaintiff is in the "zone of danger." The zone of danger refers to the dangerous area created by the negligence of the defendant. The plaintiff must be in the zone of danger, which unreasonably threatens the physical safety of the plaintiff. For example, a plaintiff's distress is from a physical injury caused by the defendant, or the plaintiff witnessed a severe injury or death of a close family member caused by the defendant.

Liability may relate to the delivery of medical services because medical services can involve life-and-death situations that may induce mental pain, suffering, and anguish. An example seen in many cases is when a parent witnesses the horrific death of a child caused by the defendant. Case law varies on whether the parent must fear for their own safety as a result of the negligence of the medical professional.

Intentional Torts

A tort is a breach or violation of a duty (responsibility) that is imposed on one person in relation to another. Similar to the legal doctrine of liability, technologists owe a duty to patients, physicians, and all other health care professionals. Of the many established torts, technologists need to be familiar with the intentional torts. *Intentional torts require the defendant to have an intent to cause harm and may be either specific or general intent.* Specific intent is when the defendant intends their actions to bring about a specific harm. In contrast, general intent is when the defendant knew to a substantial certainty that their actions would cause harm to another. Intent may also be inferred from a person's conduct or speech. The intentional torts discussed in this section are battery, assault, false imprisonment, and intentional infliction of emotional distress.

Battery

Battery is an *intentional harmful or offensive contact to the plaintiff's person.* Harmful or offensive contact may be as simple as nonconsented touching of another person. The plaintiff's person encompasses anything connected or attached to the plaintiff's body (eg, a hat or purse). In *Fisher v. Carrousel Motor Hotel*, the issue in the case was whether a plaintiff may recover for battery even though he was not physically touched by the defendant.[56] The case arose when the defendant's employee seized a plate from the hand of an African American and shouted "a Negro could not be served in the club."[57] The plaintiff sought damages for assault and battery.[58] The court held that the "intentional grabbing of plaintiff's plate constituted a battery. The intentional snatching of an object from one's hand is as clearly an offensive invasion of his person as would be an actual contact with the body."[59] The court further stated that "it is not necessary to touch the plaintiff's body or even his clothing; knocking or snatching anything from plaintiff's hand or touching anything connected with his person, when done in an offensive manner, is sufficient."[60]

Applying the concept of battery to health care leads to one of the most quoted statements regarding medical battery.[61] Justice Cardozo said: "Every human being of adult years and sound mind has a right to determine what shall be done with his own body; and a surgeon who performs an operation without his patient's consent commits … [battery], for which he is liable in damages."[62] Lack of consent (see Consent section) is an essential element of battery.[63] A diagnostic exam performed without the patient's consent may be considered battery.[64]

Some courts have applied a 2-standard test to determine medical battery: (1) Was the *patient aware* of the procedure or diagnostic operation? And (2) if so, did the *patient consent*?[65] Generally, this means that the patient knew and understood they were undergoing a CT exam and the general details of the exam prior to signing the consent form. Further, the administration or injection of drugs (eg, contrast media) against the patient's will may be battery.[66] It is important to note that the ASRT practice standards consider the use of peripherally inserted central catheter (PICC) lines or implanted ports as being within the scope of practice for technologists.[67] A technologist could use a PICC line to inject contrast media.

Another situation in which a battery could arise is if a patient retracts consent for an exam. In *Coulter v. Thomas,* an automatic blood pressure cuff was placed on the patient's arm before surgery.[68] The first time the blood pressure cuff inflated, the patient felt "extreme pain, began to sweat and tremble, and demanded the cuff to be removed."[69] The cuff inflated a second time, and she demanded that the cuff be removed.[70] The cuff was finally removed after it inflated again.[71] The blood pressure cuff was removed prior to surgery.[72] It was discovered that the blood vessels in the arm on which the blood pressure cuff was placed had hemorrhaged and blood had collected around the patient's median nerve, causing her severe and permanent injury.[73] The hemorrhage occurred below the elbow, but the cuff was placed above the elbow.[74] The patient brought a claim of battery, arguing that she expressly revoked consent to use the cuff and demanded that it be removed.[75] The court determined that in order to constitute a withdrawal of consent after the exam has begun, 2 elements are required:

1. The patient must act or use language which can be subject to no other inference and which must be unquestioned responses

from a clear and rational mind. These actions and utterances of the patient must be such as to leave no room for doubt in the minds of reasonable men that in view of all the circumstances consent was actually withdrawn.

2. When medical treatments or examinations occurring with the patient's consent are proceeding in a manner requiring bodily contact by the physician with the patient and consent to the contact is revoked, it must be medically feasible for the doctor to desist in the treatment or examination at that point without the cessation being detrimental to the patient's health or life from a medical viewpoint.[76]

The court determined that the patient satisfied both elements because she used very clear and specific language in demanding that the blood pressure cuff be removed.[77] The patient testified that she said, "Take it [the blood pressure cuff] off. I can't stand it," after the first inflation.[78]

It is important that technologists pay attention to the patient's wishes. As the court in *Coulter v. Thomas* determined, the patient must make a clear statement that they wish to stop the exam, and it must be feasible to stop without harm to the patient. If a patient uses clear and specific language that they refuse to continue with an exam, the technologist should obey the wishes of the patient and stop the exam as soon as possible. Further, a patient may terminate consent at any time. As stated in the ASRT practice standards, the technologist should inform the patient of the consequences of not completing the exam. If the patient decides to continue with the exam, they have given consent to continue and the elements of battery are not satisfied.

Assault

Assault is an intentional act by the defendant that creates a reasonable apprehension of immediate harmful or offensive contact to the plaintiff's person. It may also be considered an attempted battery. The plaintiff must have knowledge of defendant's act and a reasonable expectation that it will result in harmful or offensive contact. Also, words or threats alone are usually not enough, unless in coordination with an overt act (ie, clenching fists).

Assault and Battery Example Examples of circumstances where assault and battery could occur in the medical provider-patient setting are as follows: "1) when a physician *performs a procedure other than that for which consent was granted;* 2) when a physician performs a procedure *without obtaining any consent* from the patient; and 3) when the physician *realizes that the patient does not understand* what the procedure entails."[79] The court in *Pallacovitch v. Waterbury Hospital* applied this physician standard to a technician (phlebotomist) who performed a routine blood draw. This standard may further be applied to CT technologists. Proper patient education and consent to the exam are important to avoid an allegation of battery.

The ASRT practice standards require the technologist to verify that the patient consented (see Consent and Informed

Consent sections) to the exam and "fully understands its risks, benefits, alternatives, and follow-up."[80] The requested exam is to be verified for appropriateness before the exam begins. The technologist is to further verify that "written or informed consent has been obtained." The technologist is to explain each step of the exam to the patient and ask for cooperation of the patient.

All patients must be positioned for CT exams. The technologist must obtain consent before touching the patient. It is good practice to ask the patient if you may position them by touching them and to explain why. Patients need to be informed and consent to each step of the exam. As stated in the ASRT practice standards, patients need to be immobilized for the exam. Immobilization is necessary to restrict patient movement and provide good-quality diagnostic images. Just as when positioning the patient, the technologist must obtain consent before touching the patient. Technologists may use straps, sandbags, and sponges to immobilize the patient, especially the anatomic area of interest; however, it is important that the patient is comfortable. If the patient becomes upset and refuses to continue the exam, the technologist must stop the exam. It is good practice to remove the patient from the bore of the CT unit and discuss why they wish to stop before removing the immobilizing items, unless it is an emergency.

False Imprisonment

False imprisonment is an act or omission to act by the defendant that restrains or confines the plaintiff to a bounded area. The restraint or confinement need not be physical; threats of force may be enough. Also, the duration of restraint or confinement need not be long; a brief confinement may suffice. The plaintiff must be aware of the confinement or harmed by it. The plaintiff must not have a reasonable means of escape from the bounded area.

A patient is restrained once they are positioned, immobilized, and placed in the bore of the CT unit. The restraint of the patient must be performed with patient consent and justification. Consent applies to false imprisonment just as it did with battery. The technologist must respect the wishes of the patient. Immobilization of the patient is justified so that good diagnostic images may be obtained; however, the patient should be comfortable.

Once positioned, immobilized, and placed in the bore of the CT unit, patients know that they are confined. Prior to entering the bore of the CT unit, the technologist should inform the patient, in a professional manner, about the confining nature of the exam and how to communicate with the technologist during the exam. Also, the technologist should inform the patient that they, as the technologist performing the exam, will be continuously monitoring the exam. After placing the patient in the bore of the CT unit, the technologist should assess the patient and talk to the patient. This will reduce anxiety and lead to a better exam. It is important to note that the patient has consented to this confinement but may withdraw or refuse at any time.

Positioned and immobilized patients who are in the bore of the CT unit cannot easily remove themselves. Patients will rely on the technologist to remove them from the bore of the CT unit and to remove immobilizing devices. Ignoring a patient may lead to the patient attempting to extract themselves from the bore, which could lead to injury and may constitute false imprisonment. Once again, the technologist should respect the wishes of the patient. In addition, the technologist should assess and monitor the patient's physical, mental, and emotional status throughout the exam.

Intentional Infliction of Emotional Distress

Intentional infliction of emotional distress is intentional or reckless, extreme, and outrageous conduct by the defendant that causes the plaintiff to suffer severe emotional distress. Courts require the defendant's conduct to meet the high threshold of outrageous conduct. Outrageous conduct is conduct that exceeds all bounds of decency in society, and the plaintiff must suffer severe emotional distress as a result of the conduct.

Bystander Claim of Emotional Distress

A bystander may claim emotional distress if the bystander is closely related to the person physically injured or killed by the defendant's conduct. The defendant's actions may be negligent (see Negligent Infliction of Emotional Distress section) or intentional (see Intentional Infliction of Emotional Distress section). In addition, the plaintiff must witness the injury-causing event. For example, a father may bring a bystander claim of emotional distress after witnessing the death of a child if the child was struck and killed by a car in the father's presence.

Misrepresentation

Misrepresentation is the intent to deceive someone by making false statements or concealing important facts. Technologists could misrepresent themselves as medical doctors. For example, after completing an exam, a technologist tells a patient that the patient has cancer. The technologist may be liable for misrepresentation because the technologist concealed that they were a technologist, not a physician, and acted outside the scope of practice for a technologist.

Defamation

Defamation is harm to the plaintiff's reputation caused by a statement made by the defendant to a third person that concerns the plaintiff. If the statement is a matter of public concern or involves a public figure or official, then the plaintiff must prove that the statement was false and the defendant was at fault. Technologists must not make false statements about patients or coworkers. Statements may quickly spread and harm the reputation of the plaintiff. In addition, social media allows for the quick dissemination of information, regardless of whether the information is true or false.

Defenses to Intentional Torts

The first defense is that the plaintiff did not meet the elements, but if the plaintiff did meet the elements, then the defendant may offer several defenses. In addition to consent, discussed in the next section, the defendant can argue that the plaintiff gave informed consent to perform the exam or procedure (see Informed Consent section).

Consent

Consent is a defense to all intentional torts. Consent is approval or permission voluntarily given by a competent person to the defendant's otherwise tortious conduct. Patients or patient representatives must consent to the CT exam, venipuncture, and administration of contrast agents after being informed. The ASRT practice standards require technologists to verify and document that the patient consents to the exam prior to the exam. Technologists may be liable for an intentional tort if the patient retracts consent and the exam continues or if the patient has not given consent in the first instance. If a patient refuses the exam or retracts consent, it is good practice for a technologist to inform their supervisor and document the incident.

Consent may not be necessary in emergency situations, where consent may not be obtained and medical treatment is crucial. In emergency situations where consent has not been obtained, technologists should follow the written policy of their employer and direction of the attending physician and/or attending radiologist. Hospitals may have internal emergency policies regarding consent. In addition, surrogates (eg, family members) may consent for the patient to undergo the exam. Once again, technologists should follow the written policy of their employer and direction of the attending physician and/or attending radiologist.

OVEREXPOSURE CASE EXAMPLES

Example 1 (Figure 3–1)

In 2008, a 2.5-year-old boy was overexposed to ionizing radiation during a CT exam.[81] The child was taken to the emergency department after falling out of bed and having trouble moving his head.[82] A CT exam of his cervical spine was ordered by the emergency department physician.[83] A normal exam would have taken only a few minutes to complete.[84] This CT exam took 68 minutes, and the child was exposed to 151 scans of the same area.[85] After a few hours, the child "developed a bright red ring around his head from the massive radiation overdose."[86] Radiation injury specialist, Dr Fred Mettler, believed "the most likely medical effect on the boy will be the formation of cataracts, but the other parts of the body that were exposed, the salivary glands, brain, and eyes, could also be affected in the future."[87] The technologist who performed the CT exam was fired, and her license was suspended.[88] The parents of the child filed a lawsuit that claimed negligence and medical battery by

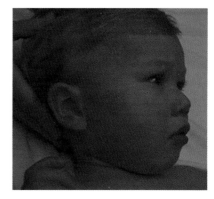

FIGURE 3–1. Note the bright red ring around the head of the child due to overexposure. (Image courtesy of Roth family attorney Don Stockett.)

the technologist and hospital.[89] The hospital and child's family reached a confidential settlement.[90]

Example 2

On October 8, 2009, US the Food and Drug Administration (FDA) issued a notification regarding radiation overexposure of 206 patients who had CT brain perfusion exams at one medical center over the course of 18 months.[91] CT brain perfusion exams are used to assist in stroke diagnosis and treatment.[92] Due to incorrect settings at the CT scanner console, patients received approximately 8 times the expected dose of radiation for that procedure.[93] Of the 206 overexposed patients, approximately 40% of them reported some hair loss due to the high radiation dose.[94]

On October 26, 2010, after continued investigation, the FDA knew of "approximately 385 patients from six hospitals who were exposed to excess radiation during CT brain perfusion" exams.[95] Again, some overexposed patients reported hair loss or skin redness after the exam.[96] Overexposure to radiation may go undetected and unreported when the radiation dose is high but not quite high enough for observable signs of radiation injury.[97] Over time, excess radiation may increase the risk of long-term effects, such as cancer.[98]

The CT scanners involved in the overexposure were manufactured by 2 different manufacturers.[99] The FDA found that the manufacturers did not violate any FDA laws or regulations.[100] Further, the scanners were evaluated, and it was found the scanners did not produce an overexposure when "used according to the manufacturers' specifications."[101] The FDA investigation revealed that technologist information and training would improve safety and decrease the probability of overexposure.[102]

DOCUMENTATION

Technologists need to document "information about patient care, the procedure, and the final outcome" because "clear and precise documentation is essential for continuity of care, accuracy of care and quality of assurance."[103] Generally, the technologist should document all pertinent information. For example, the technologist should:

- Verify the patient's medical history
- Note important facts in the patient's medical history (eg, implant records, labs)
- Verify and record pertinent exam information
- Document pertinent exam details in the patient's medical record (following the employer's policies and procedures)
- Document whether contrast media was administered and, if so, specifically document:
  - Injection site
  - Type of needle
  - Gauge of needle
  - Type of contrast administered
  - Amount administered
  - Whether it was hand injected or power injected
  - Flow rate
  - Any complications

This list is not exhaustive, and the technologist should follow their employer's policies and procedures. Generally, it is good to document all information that the technologist believes is important because if a supervisor, an attorney, or anyone else has a question about an exam, then they may review the technologist's notes.

HEALTH INSURANCE PORTABILITY AND ACCOUNTABILITY ACT AND HEALTH INFORMATION TECHNOLOGY FOR ECONOMIC AND CLINICAL HEALTH ACT

The Health Insurance Portability and Accountability Act (HIPAA) is a federal law that all technologists need to understand, particularly the HIPAA Privacy Rule. It is important to note that HIPAA is only one of many complex confidentiality laws.

The Health Information Technology for Economic and Clinical Health (HITECH) Act revised HIPAA and amended enforcement regulations. The Privacy Rule applies to most health care plans and providers that use electronic transmission of protected patient health information. The Privacy Rule limited the disclosure or use of someone's protected health information by a covered entity. The protected health information must be disclosed to (1) individuals or authorized representatives if they specifically request access or an accounting of their health information and (2) the Department of Health and Human Services when completing a compliance review, enforcement action, or investigation. Disclosure or use of protected health information without the person's authorization is permitted for payment, treatment, or health care operations. Any other purposes require the covered entity to obtain the person's written authorization.

The covered entity must make an effort to only allow the minimum disclosure and use of protected health information. Health care employees should be provided only the necessary information to complete their job. Covered entities, such as hospitals and clinics, also limit employee access to patient information, where they only have sufficient information to perform their job functions and roles. A common example of unlawful disclosure and use is when a third party overhears employees discussing a patient. The third party would have received access to patient information that they did not have authorization to receive.

The covered entity may disclose protected health information without authorization when required by law (eg, victims of abuse, neglect, or domestic violence; law enforcement purposes; judicial and administrative proceedings); to prevent or control disease, disability, or injury; for authorized health oversight activities; when decedents (eg, funeral directors, coroners, medical examiners) are involved; to facilitate organ or tissue donation; when research is involved; to prevent or reduce a serious and imminent threat to someone; for essential government functions; and for workers' compensation.

Limited data sets may also be released when direct identifiers of individuals, household members, relatives, and employers have been removed. Direct identifiers include the following:

1. Names
2. Postal address information, other than town or city, state, and zip code
3. Telephone numbers
4. Fax numbers
5. Email addresses
6. Social Security numbers
7. Medical record numbers
8. Health plan beneficiary numbers
9. Account numbers
10. Certificate/license numbers
11. Vehicle identifiers and serial numbers, including license plate numbers
12. Device identifiers and serial numbers
13. Web universal resource locators (URLs)
14. Internet protocol (IP) address numbers
15. Biometric identifiers, including finger and voice prints
16. Full face photographic images and any comparable images[104]

The limited data set information may be used for research, public health purposes, or health care operations. The covered entity should obtain satisfactory assurance, in the form of a data use agreement, that the limited data set recipient will only use or disclose the protected health information for limited purposes.[105] It is important for technologists to read their employers' HIPAA policies.

AMERICAN REGISTRY OF RADIOLOGIC TECHNOLOGISTS STANDARD OF ETHICS

The first part of the American Registry of Radiologic Technologists (ARRT) Standard of Ethics is the Code of Ethics, which is a guide of "professional conduct as it relates to patients, healthcare consumers, employers, colleagues, and other members of the healthcare team."[106] The Code of Ethics is aspirational, with the intent of "maintaining a high level of ethical conduct and in providing for the protection, safety, and comfort of patients."[107]

1. The Registered Technologist *acts in a professional manner*, responds to patient needs, and supports colleagues and associates in providing quality patient care.

2. The Registered Technologist acts to advance the principal objective of the profession to *provide services to humanity* with full respect for the dignity of mankind.

3. The Registered Technologist delivers patient care and service unrestricted by the concerns of personal attributes or the nature of the disease or illness, and without discrimination on the basis of race, color, creed, religion, national origin, sex, marital status, status with regard to public assistance, familial status, disability, sexual orientation, gender identity, veteran status, age, or any other legally protected basis.

4. The Registered Technologist practices technology founded upon theoretical knowledge and concepts, *uses equipment and accessories consistent with the purposes for which they were designed*, and *employs procedures and techniques appropriately*.

5. The Registered Technologist assesses situations; exercises care, discretion, and judgment; assumes responsibility for professional decisions; and *acts in the best interest of the patient*.

6. The Registered Technologist acts as an agent through observation and communication to *obtain pertinent information for the physician* to aid in the diagnosis and treatment of the patient and recognizes that *interpretation and diagnosis are outside the scope of practice* for the profession.

7. The Registered Technologist uses equipment and accessories, employs techniques and procedures, *performs services in accordance with an accepted standard of practice*, and demonstrates expertise in *minimizing radiation exposure* to the patient, self, and other members of the healthcare team.

8. The Registered Technologist *practices ethical conduct* appropriate to the profession and protects the patient's right to quality radiologic technology care.

9. The Registered Technologist *respects confidences* entrusted in the course of professional practice, *respects the patient's right to privacy*, and reveals confidential information only as required by law or to protect the welfare of the individual or the community.

10. The Registered Technologist continually strives to improve knowledge and skills by *participating in continuing education and professional activities*, sharing knowledge with colleagues, and investigating new aspects of professional practice.

11. The Registered Technologist *refrains from the use of illegal drugs and/or legally controlled substances which result in impairment of professional judgement* and/or ability to practice radiologic technology with reasonable skill and safety to patients.[108]

The Rules of Ethics compose the second part of the Standard of Ethics.[109] The rules are mandatory standards of minimal professional conduct for registered technologists and applicants.[110] The rules are intended to promote safety, protection, and comfort for patients and are enforceable.[111] Registered technologists are required to notify the ARRT of any ethics violation within 30 days of the occurrence or during annual renewal and registration.[112] The rules cover (1) fraud or deceptive practices; (2) subversion; (3) unprofessional conduct and scope of practice; (4) fitness to practice; (5) improper management of patient records; (6) violation of state or federal law or regulatory rule; and (7) duty to report.[113] For a comprehensive explanation of each rule, please review the ARRT Standards of Ethics.

Bibliography

American Hospital Association. Patient Bill of Rights. Accessed February 2022. https://www.americanpatient.org/aha-patients-bill-of-rights/

American Law Institute. *Restatement of the Law Second, Torts*. American Law Institute; 1979.

American Registry of Radiologic Technologists. *ARRT Standards of Ethics*. September 1, 2021. Accessed August 31, 2022. https://assets-us-01.kc-usercontent.com/406ac8c6-58e8-00b3-e3c1-0c312965deb2/eac1b19c-a45a-4e65-917b-922115ff2c15/arrt-standards-of-ethics.pdf

American Society of Radiologic Technologists. *The ASRT Practice Standards for Medical Imaging and Radiation Therapy*. June 20, 2021. Accessed August 31, 2022. https://www.asrt.org/docs/default-source/practice-standards/asrt-practice-standards-for-medical-imaging-and-radiation-therapy.pdf?sfvrsn=de532d0_24

Boumil MM, Elias CE, Moes DB. *Medical Liability: In a Nutshell*. 2nd ed. West; 2003.

Bryant v. Oakpointe Villa Nursing Ctr., 684 N.W.2d 864, 871 (Mich. 2004).

Byrne v. Boadle, 159 Eng. Rep. 299 (Ex. 1863).

Caldwell v. Vanderbilt U., M2012-00328-COA-R3CV, 2013 WL 655239, slip op. at 1 (Tenn. App. 2013); *Brief of Defendants/Appellee the Vanderbilt U. d/b/a Vanderbilt U. Medical Center*, 2011 WL 10549728 (Tenn. Cir. Ct.).

Colombini et al. v. Westchester County Healthcare Corporation et al., 2002 WL 34160371 (N.Y. Sup.).

Colombini v. Westchester County Health Care Corp., 899 N.Y.S.2d 58, 2009 NY Slip Op 51555(U).

Coulter v. Thomas, 33S.W.3d 522, 523 (Ky. 2000).

Defense Against a Prima Facie Case § 14:48, Intentional Infliction (Rev. ed., March 2014).

Defense Against a Prima Facie Case § 14:49, Negligent Infliction (Rev. ed., March 2014).

Furrow BR, Greaney TL, Johnson SH, Jost TS, Schwartz RL. *Law and Health Care Quality, Patient Safety, and Medical Liability*. West Academic Publishing; 2013.

Garner BA, ed. *Black's Law Dictionary*. 9th ed. West Group; 2009.

Harris DM. *Healthcare Law and Ethics: Issues for the Age of Managed Care*. Health Administration Press; 1999.

Pallacovitch v. Waterbury Hosp., No. CV126013332, 2012 WL 3667310 (Conn. Super. Ct. Aug. 3, 2012).

Trinckes JJ Jr. *The Definitive Guide to Complying with the HIPPA/ HITECH Privacy and Security Rules*. CRC Press; 2013.

Twerski AD, Henderson JA, Wendel WB. *Torts: Cases and Materials*. Wolters Kluwer Law & Business; 2012.

USA.gov. Branches of the U.S. Government. Accessed August 31, 2022. https://www.usa.gov/branches-of-government

US State Courts. *Federal Rules of Civil Procedure*. December 1, 2020. Accessed August 31, 2022. https://www.uscourts.gov/sites/default/files/federal_rules_of_civil_procedure_-_december_2020_0.pdf

Ybarra v. Spangard, 25 Cal. 2d 486, 487, 154 P.2d 687 (1944).

Yeazell SC. *Civil Procedure*. 8th ed. Wolters Kluwer Law & Business; 2012.

References

1. Duszak R Jr, Berlin L, Ellenbogen PH. Stability and infrequency of radiologic technologist malpractice payments: an analysis of the National Practitioner Data Bank. *J Am Coll Radiol*. 2010;7:705. The NPDB is maintained by the Department of Health and Human Services.

2. *Id.*

3. *Id.*

4. *Id.* at 706. Health care providers are categorized according to their state license types. *Id.* Applicable categories include nuclear medicine technologists, radiologic technologist, and x-ray technician or operator. *Id.* These 4 categories were grouped together for the study. *Id.*

5. *Id.*

6. *Id.* Thirty of the 155 cases listed in the NPDB were reported as malpractice act or omission, and 24 cases were reported as allegation not otherwise specified. *Id.* at 707. A third of the 131 cases listed in a specific and identifiable category were reported as diagnostic errors, which included "failure to diagnose and wrong or misdiagnosis." *Id.* Another third of the 131 cases were reported as "improper technique; failure to monitor; failure to conform with regulation state, or rule; and improper conduct." *Id.*

7. *Id.* at 706.

8. *Id.*

9. *Id.* Payments were adjusted to 2008 dollars by using the Bureau of Labor Statistics Consumer Price Index. *Id.*

10. *Id.* at 706-707.

11. *Id.* at 707.

12. *Id.* at 708. The nation's population increased from 252,980,941 to 304,059,724, representing a 20% increase. *Id.* The government's labor statistics indicated that from 1988 to 2008, the number of radiologic technologists increased from 132,000 to 214,700, representing a 63% increase. *Id.* The American Registry of Radiologic Technologists estimated that the actual number of technologists in 2008 was 278,415. *Id.*

13. *Id.*

14. *Id.*

15. *Id.* at 709.

16. *Id.* at 708.

17. *Id.*

18. *Id.*

19. *Id.*

20. *Id.* at 709.

21. *Id.* Here, borrowed servant may be defined as "[a] physician … who borrows [temporarily] another's employee may be liable for the employee's negligent acts if he acquires the same right of control over the employee as originally possessed by a lending employer." *Id.*

22. *Id.* The Oregon Supreme Court held in a case involving a misdiagnosis that while technologists are skilled in taking x-rays, they are not experts in determining whether the images are sufficient. *Id.* The radiologist is responsible for reading the images and determining whether the images are sufficient. *Id.*

23. See, generally, American Society of Radiologic Technologists. *The ASRT Practice Standards for Medical Imaging and Radiation Therapy*. June 20, 2021. https://www.asrt.org/docs/default-source/practice-standards/asrt-practice-standards-for-medical-imaging-and-radiation-therapy.pdf?sfvrsn=de532d0_24

24. *Id.* at PS 3.

25. *Id.*

26. *Id.*

27. *Id.*

28. Leahy MCM. *Radiation Overexposure From CT Scans and Resulting Cancer Risk*. 127 Am. Jur. Trials 395 (originally published in 2012). *Emphasis added.*

29. *Bryant v. Oakpointe Villa Nursing Ctr.*, 684 N.W.2d 864, 871 (Mich. 2004).

30. *Id. Emphasis added.*

31. *Id.*

32. *Id.*

33. *Caldwell v. Vanderbilt U.*, M2012-00328-COA-R3CV, 2013 WL 655239 (Tenn. App. 2013); *Brief of Defendants/Appellee the Vanderbilt U. d/b/a Vanderbilt U. Medical Center*, 2011 WL 10549728 (Tenn. Cir. Ct.).

34. James AE Jr, ed. *Legal Medicine With Special Reference to Diagnostic Imaging*. Urban & Schwarzenberg; 1980.

35. Penofsky D. *Diagnostic Radiology Malpractice Litigation*. 75 Am. Jur. Trials (2000) 55, at § 78 (May 2016 Update).

36. Actual causation.

37. Proximate causation.

38. Furrow BR, Greaney TL, Johnson SH, Jost TS, Schwartz RL. *Law and Health Care Quality, Patient Safety, and Medical Liability*. West Academic Publishing; 2013:305.

39. *Byrne v. Boadle*, 159 Eng. Rep. 299 (Ex. 1863).

40. Twerski AD, Henderson JA, Wendel WB. *Torts: Cases and Materials*. Wolters Kluwer Law & Business; 2012.

41. *Scott v. London & St. Katherine Docs Co.*, 159 Eng. Rep. 665, 667 (Ex. 1865).

42. *Toogood v. Owen J. Rogal, D.D.S., P.C.*, 824 A.2d 1140 (Pa. 2003).

43. Prosser & Keeton. (5th ed. 1995). *The Law of Torts* § 39, p. 243.

44. *Ybarra v. Spangard*, 25 Cal. 2d 486, 154 P.2d 687 (1944).

45. *Id.* at 487, 154 P.2d at 688.

46. Contributory negligence is another defense to negligence, but most states have abolished contributory negligence doctrine in favor of comparative negligence doctrine. Contributory negligence is when the plaintiff's own negligence was a part in causing the injury. In some states, this is enough to prevent the plaintiff from recovering any damages, but other states reduce the plaintiff's recoverable damages by the percent fault attributed to their own misconduct. For example, a patient (plaintiff) fails to disclose their full medical history to the technologist and suffers an injury as a result. The technologist may claim that the patient was contributory negligent by not disclosing their full medical history. The court could find the patient was 40% contributory negligent because their own negligence was a part in causing the injury and could therefore reduce their total awards by 40%.

47. Furrow B., Greaney TL, Johnson SH, Jost TS, Schwartz RL. *Law and Health Care Quality, Patient Safety, and Medical Liability*. West Academic Publishing; 2013:195.

48. *Id.*

49. *Conte v. Girard Orthopaedic Surgeons Med. Group, Inc.*, 132 Cal. Rptr. 2d 855, 859 (Cal. App. 4th Dist. 2003); *Cobbs v. Grant*, 502 P.2d 1, 7-10 (Cal. 1972); M.G. v. A. I. Dupont Hosp. for Children, 393 Fed. Appx. 884, 889 (3d Cir. Pa. 2010).

50. *Conte v. Girard Orthopaedic Surgeons Med. Group, Inc.*, 132 Cal. Rptr. 2d 855, 859 (Cal. App. 4th Dist. 2003).

51. *Id.*

52. American Society of Radiologic Technologists. *The ASRT Practice Standards for Medical Imaging and Radiation Therapy*. PS 14. June 20, 2021. https://www.asrt.org/docs/default-source/practice-standards/asrt-practice-standards-for-medical-imaging-and-radiation-therapy.pdf?sfvrsn=de532d0_24

53. *Steve Herbst v. IMI Acquisition Arlington Corp.*

54. *Reproduced with permission from Gumm vs. North Valley MRI & CT Center. 30 Trials Digest 63. Westlaw/Thomson Reuters Corporation.*

55. *Reproduced with permission from Newton, Estate of v. Botsford General Hospital; Botsford Medical Imaging PC. JVR No. 1306250010. Westlaw/Thomson Reuters Corporation.*

56. *Fisher v. Carrousel Motor Hotel*, 424 S.W.2d 627, 628 (Tex. 1967).

57. *Fisher v. Carrousel Motor Hotel*, 424 S.W.2d 627, 628-629 (Tex. 1967).

58. *Fisher v. Carrousel Motor Hotel*, 424 S.W.2d 627, 628 (Tex. 1967).

59. *Fisher v. Carrousel Motor Hotel*, 424 S.W.2d 627, 629 (Tex. 1967).

60. *Id.*

61. James AE Jr, ed. *Legal Medicine With Special Reference to Diagnostic Imaging*. Urban & Schwarzenberg; 1980.

62. *Schloendorff v. Society of New York Hospital*, 105 N.E. 92, 129-130 (N.Y. App. 1914). Justice Cardozo misstated when he said the surgeon committed an assault; the surgeon actually committed a battery. James AE Jr, ed. *Legal Medicine With Special Reference to Diagnostic Imaging*. Urban & Schwarzenberg; 1980.

63. *Vitale v. Henchey*, 24 S.W.3d 651, 658 (Ky. 2000).

64. James AE Jr, ed. *Legal Medicine With Special Reference to Diagnostic Imaging*. Urban & Schwarzenberg; 1980.

65. *Shuler v. Garrett*, 743 F.3d 170, 173 (6th Cir. 2014). *Emphasis added.* This is a federal court case and is not applicable to all state medical malpractice cases.

66. *Shuler v. Garrett*, 743 F.3d 170, 174 (6th Cir. 2014).

67. American Society of Radiologic Technologists. *The Practice Standards for Medical Imaging and Radiation Therapy Advisory Opinion Statement: Injecting Medication in Peripherally Inserted Central Catheter Lines or Ports with a Power Injector*. American Society of Radiologic Technologists; June 2018.

68. *Coulter v. Thomas*, 33 S.W.3d 522, 523 (Ky. 2000).

69. *Id.*

70. *Id.*

71. *Id.*

72. *Id.*

73. *Id.*

74. *Id.*

75. *Id.*

76. *Id.* At 524.

77. *Id.*

78. *Id.*

79. *Pallacovitch v. Waterbury Hosp.*, No. CV126013332, 2012 WL 3667310 (Conn. Super. Ct. Aug. 3, 2012), quoting *Logan v. Greenwich Hospital Assn.*, 465 A.2d 294, 298 (Conn. 1983). *Emphasis added.*

80. American Society of Radiologic Technologists. *The ASRT Practice Standards for Medical Imaging and Radiation Therapy*. June 20, 2021. https://www.asrt.org/docs/default-source/practice-standards/asrt-practice-standards-for-medical-imaging-and-radiation-therapy.pdf?sfvrsn=de532d0_24

81. Bogdanich W. Radiation overdoses point up dangers of CT scans. *The New York Times*. October 16, 2009. http://www.nytimes.com/2009/10/16/us/16radiation.html?_r=0

82. Domino D. Settlement reached in Mad River pediatric CT radiation case. *Aunt Minnie*. May 24, 2010. http://www.auntminnie.com/index.aspx?sec=ser&sub=def&pag=dis&ItemID=90713

83. *Id.*

84. Bogdanich, *supra* note 1.

85. Domino, *supra* note 2.

86. *Id.*

87. *Id.*

88. *Id.*

89. *Id.*

90. *Id.*

91. US Food and Drug Administration. Safety investigation of CT brain perfusion scans. FDA; Update November 9, 2010; and Wintermark M, Lev MH. FDA investigates the safety of brain perfusion CT. *Am J Neuroradiol*. 2010;31:2.

92. *Id.*

93. Wintermark M, Lev MH. FDA investigates the safety of brain perfusion CT. *Am J Neuroradiol.* 2010;31:2.

94. *Id.*

95. US Food and Drug Administration, *supra* note 48.

96. *Id.*

97. *Id.*

98. *Id.*

99. *Id.*

100. *Id.*

101. *Id.*

102. *Id.*

103. *Id.* at PS 40.

104. 45 CFR § 164.514(e)(2).

105. 45 CFR § 164.514(e)(4)(i).

106. Reproduced with permission from *ARRT Standards of Ethics.* September 1, 2021. © 2021 The American Registry of Radiologic Technologists.

107. *Id.*

108. *Id. Emphasis added.*

109. *Id.*

110. *Id.*

111. *Id.*

112. *Id.*

113. *Id.*

PART II

Introduction to Imaging Applications

4

Brain and Head Positioning

Proper positioning of the patient's body and, more importantly, the specific anatomic area that has been requested to be imaged are essential to providing quality images to the radiologist. Most CT procedures will be performed with the patient in the supine position. Once the patient is safely on the CT scanning table, it is suggested that the patient be positioned as straight as possible. To assist with performing this task, a review of key anatomic structures is useful. For brain and head imaging, these structures include the glabella, nasion, and mental point of the patient's face (Figure 4–1). Other anatomic structures along the midline of the patient and associated with imaging the chest, abdomen, and pelvis include the jugular notch and xiphoid process of the sternum, the umbilicus of the abdomen, and the midpoint of the pelvis (pubic symphysis) are helpful landmarks to use in ensuring that the patient is straight on the patient couch.

When imaging the brain or other head-related structures, accurate positioning of the patient's head is important so that the internal anatomic structures are symmetrically presented. From the frontal view (see Figure 4–1), key landmarks include the glabella, nasion, and mental point. Further, the interpupillary line should be perpendicular to the midsagittal plane of the patient's face. This will help to ensure there is less rotation and tilting of the internal anatomic structures and improve the comparison of left-sided versus right-sided structures. From the lateral view (Figure 4–2), key lines for alignment are the orbitomeatal line (OML) and the supraorbitomeatal line (SOML) for gantry angulation.

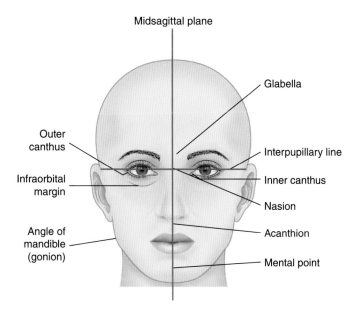

FIGURE 4–1. Frontal view showing key anatomic structures used for positioning of the head. Midline structures such as the glabella, nasion, acanthion, and mental point are used to define the midsagittal plane. Using the midline structures, align so they are straight and without rotation. The interpupillary line identifies a line between the pupils of the patient's eyes. To avoid tilt of the patient's head, when positioning, align the interpupillary line to be perpendicular to the midsagittal plane. Make sure this line is not angled. In doing so, the resultant anatomy when comparing the left side and right side should appear similar. When positioned properly, the axial images should not demonstrate any signs of rotation or tilt. (Reproduced with permission from Jones J, Long BW, Rollins JH, Smith BJ. *Merrill's Atlas of Radiographic Positioning and Procedures*, Vol 2. 13th ed. Elsevier; 2016.)

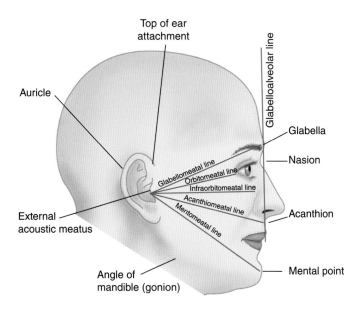

FIGURE 4–2. Lateral view showing key anatomic structures used to assist in positioning the head for a CT exam. If possible, position the patient's head with the orbitomeatal line (OML) perpendicular to the table. The OML is defined as a line between the outer canthus of the eye to the external auditory meatus (EAM). This line may also be referred to as the outer canthomeatal line or just the canthomeatal line (CML). To decrease the chance of excessive radiation exposure to the lens of the eye, the gantry of the CT unit should be angled along the supraorbitomeatal line (SOML). (Reproduced with permission from Jones J, Long BW, Rollins JH, Smith BJ. *Merrill's Atlas of Radiographic Positioning and Procedures*, Vol 2. 13th ed. Elsevier; 2016.)

5

Routine Brain

INDICATIONS

Headache, seizures, syncope, altered mental status, intracranial hemorrhage, suspected mass or tumor, neurologic defects, hydrocephalus, brain herniation, acute trauma, postoperative brain surgery, drug toxicity, and if the patient is unable to undergo an MRI due to a contraindication.

IMAGING APPLICATIONS

Patient/Part Positioning

Position the patient supine and headfirst in the gantry. Position the head straight on the table with the orbitomeatal line (OML) perpendicular to the table. Align the midsagittal plane of the patient's head so there is no rotation. Adjust the interpupillary line so it is perpendicular to the midline sagittal plane of the patient's head. If the patient is kyphotic ask the patient to pull their chin down toward their chest. This will help with tube alignment along the supraorbitomeatal line (SOML). See the Chapter 4.

Breathing Instructions

Shallow breathing.

Scan Range

Caudocranial from the floor of the calvarium to the vertex.

Gantry Angulation

Parallel to the SOML. The SOML may also be called the glabellomeatal line; however, the preferred term is the SOML. The SOML should be used to reduce radiation to the lens of the eye. See Figures 5–1 to 5–3.

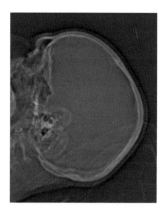

FIGURE 5–1. Lateral scout of the head used to align the slice overlay before imaging.

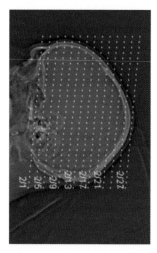

FIGURE 5–2. Lateral scout view with slice overlay. Notice the initial slice along the supraorbital meatal line (SOML). This angulation greatly reduces radiation exposure to the lens of the eye.

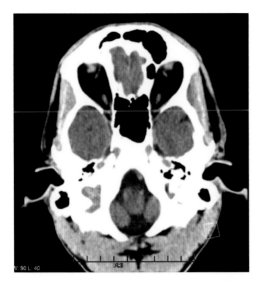

FIGURE 5–3. Initial image of the brain exam. Note the frontal lobes of brain in the frontal or anterior fossa and the temporal lobes of brain in the temporal or middle fossa areas. In the posterior fossa area are the cerebellar tonsils lateral to the medulla oblongata. This CT image demonstrates good symmetry with no signs of rotation or tilt. Further, radiation exposure to the lens of the eyes is greatly reduced.

Note: Performing CT exams of the brain in multidetector CT units where the gantry cannot tilt increases the risk of exposing the lens of the patient's eyes to a harmful amount of radiation.

Slice Thickness

Usually, from the floor of the calvarium through the fossa region (infratentorial), 5-mm slice thickness is acquired. Once through the fossa region (supratentorial), 8-mm slice thickness is sufficient for most diagnostic requirements.

Table Movement

Caudocranial.

Reconstruction Kernel/Algorithm

Standard and bone algorithms.

Window Level (WL)/Window Width (WW)

Approximate setting for:

- Brain tissue: +40 HU = WL; +100 HU = WW
- Bone window: +300 HU = WL; +1500 HU = WW

SPECIAL CONSIDERATIONS

Multiplanar Reconstruction (MPR)

Using an axial image, position the slice overlay to produce coronal MPR images (Figure 5–4) and position vertical to produce sagittal MPR images. For sagittal images, use an odd number of

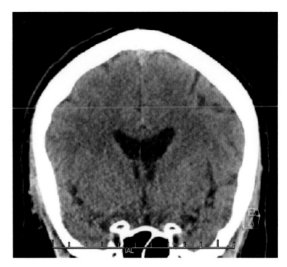

FIGURE 5–4. Coronal MPR.

slices and align the middle slice along the midline to produce a midline sagittal image of the brain (Figure 5–5) and brainstem.

Contrast Media

If intravenous (IV) contrast is needed, for adults with an acceptable glomerular filtration rate, administer (GFR) 100 mL total volume at 2 mL/s. Consult the reading radiologist for pediatric dose.

Radiation Reduction Option

Angle parallel to the SOML to reduce radiation exposure to the lens of the eyes. The first image of a CT brain should appear similar to the one in Figure 5–3. Note the symmetrical positioning of the brain showing 4 areas of brain tissue: frontal lobes; left and right temporal lobes; and brainstem with cerebellar tonsils. This positioning demonstrates imaging of the brain without exposing the lens of the eyes to unnecessary radiation.

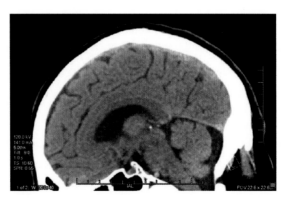

FIGURE 5–5. Midline sagittal MPR.

6

CTA Brain: Circle of Willis

INDICATIONS

CT angiography (CTA) of the cerebral arteries. Indications include occlusions, thrombosis, carotid artery stenosis, aneurysms, and vascular malformations.

IMAGING APPLICATIONS

Patient/Part Positioning

Position the patient supine and headfirst in the gantry. Position the head straight on the table with the orbitomeatal line (OML) perpendicular to the table. Align the midsagittal plane of the patient's head so there is no rotation. Adjust the interpupillary line so it is perpendicular to the midline sagittal plane of the patient's head. The patient's arms are positioned by their side. See Chapter 4.

Breathing Instructions

Breathing is suspended.

Scan Range

Caudocranial from the foramen magnum to the vertex (Figures 6–1 and 6–2). If combining the carotids with the cerebral arteries, then scan from the mid-chest (aortic arch) to the vertex.

Gantry Angulation

Gantry angulation is 0 degrees.

Slice Thickness

Thin-section imaging will produce better spatial resolution.

Table Movement

Spiral mode.

Reconstruction Kernel/Algorithm

A sharp reconstruction kernel may allow better visualization than a smooth kernel.

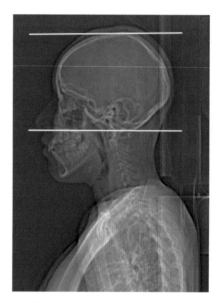

FIGURE 6–1. Lateral scout with slice alignment and scan range extending from the foramen magnum to the vertex.

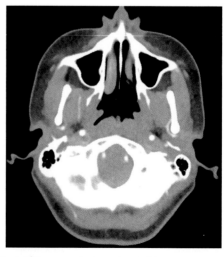

FIGURE 6–2. Axial image at the lower level of the scan range.

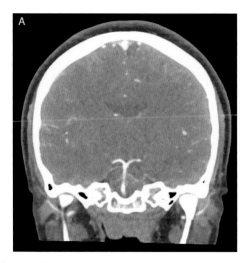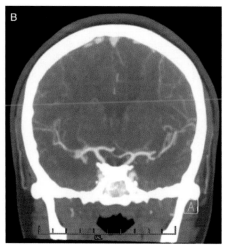

FIGURE 6–3. (A and B) Coronal MIP images showing basilar artery and superior sagittal sinus (SSS)A. Middle cerebral arteries are seen in B.

Window Level (WL)/Window Width (WW)

Approximate setting for:

- Brain tissue: +40 HU = WL; +100 HU = WW
- Bone window: +300 HU = WL; +1500 HU = WW
- Coronal and sagittal maximum intensity projection (MIP): +80 HU = WL; +700 HU = WW

Contrast Media

Intravenous (IV) contrast is used to enhance the blood vessels of the brain. The brain is supplied by 2 sets of vessels. The anterior circulation (ie, common carotid artery) and the posterior circulation (ie, vertebral arteries) combine to form the circle of Willis (COW).

Place the bolus tracking region of interest (ROI) in the descending portion of the aortic arch. The threshold is set at 100 HU with a minimal scan delay. IV contrast is injected at a rate of 4 to 5 mL/s. A saline chaser follows to allow all contrast to clear the connecting tube and enter the patient.

SPECIAL CONSIDERATIONS

Multiplanar Reconstruction (MPR)

Using an axial image, position the slice overlay to produce coronal MPR images (Figures 6–3A and 6–3B) and position vertical to produce sagittal MPR images (Figure 6–4).

Radiation Reduction

No suggestions.

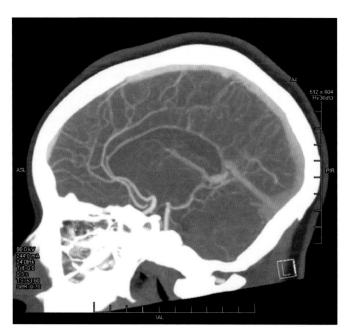

FIGURE 6–4. Sagittal MIP image along the midline showing anterior cerebral arteries, basilar artery, and the superior sagittal sinus merging with the straight sinus at the confluence of sinuses before continuing laterally as the lateral (transverse) sinuses.

7

Trauma Brain

INDICATIONS

Acute trauma such as in the case of a motor vehicle accident, projectile injury, and other forms of blunt trauma to the head.

IMAGING APPLICATIONS

Patient/Part Positioning

See instructions in Chapter 5.

Scan Range

See instructions in Chapter 5. If multiplanar reconstruction (MPR) and 3-dimensional reconstruction techniques such as shaded surface display (SSD) are requested, the scan range may be adjusted to begin at the base of the occipital bone and extend to the vertex of the skull (Figure 7–1). Note: Left-to-right midline shift.

Gantry Angulation

See instructions in Chapter 5. If MPR and SSD techniques are requested, a 0-degree gantry angulation is used.

As a suggestion, if beam hardening artifact in the posterior fossa region impedes image quality of the brainstem and cerebellum, a 0-degree gantry angulation may be helpful in improving image quality. Repeat the lateral scout and set the scan range from the foramen of magnum through the petrous portions (ridges) of the temporal bones.

Slice Thickness

See instructions in Chapter 5. If MPR and SSD techniques are requested, use thin-slice reconstruction.

Table Movement

See instructions in Chapter 5. If MPR and SSD techniques are requested, use helical mode.

Reconstruction Kernel/Algorithm

Standard/bone algorithms.

Window Level (WL)/Window Width (WW)

Approximate setting for:

- Brain tissue: +40 HU = WL; +100 HU = WW
- Bone window: +300 HU = WL; +1500 HU = WW

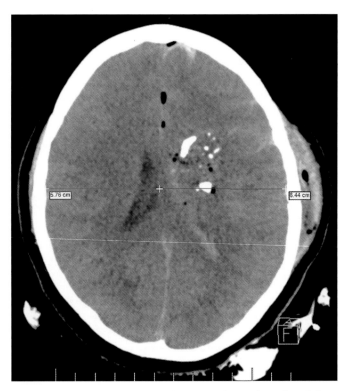

FIGURE 7–1. Helical axial CT image showing a left-to-right midline shift. Note the measurements of 6.44 cm from left to midline and 5.76 cm from right to midline. This results in an approximate left-to-right midline shift of 0.7 cm. Using the region of interest (ROI) is helpful in measuring the CT number (mean) and the standard deviation (SD) of tissues such as bone fragments, fresh blood, and air.

SPECIAL CONSIDERATIONS

- Multiplanar Reconstruction (MPR): Using an axial image, position the slice overlay to produce coronal MPR images (Figure 7–2) and position vertically to produce sagittal MPR images (Figures 7–3A and 7–3B). For the sagittal images, use an odd number of slices and align the middle slice along the midline to produce a midline sagittal image of the brain and brainstem.
- Three-dimensional SSD and (volume rendering) (VR) data reconstruction of the brain and skull may be helpful in further evaluation of the bony structures and vascular structures.

Contrast Media

Consult the radiologist.

Radiation Reduction

See instructions in Chapter 5. If MPR and SSD techniques are requested, helical mode is used to scan from the base of the

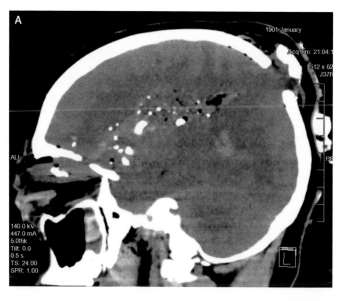

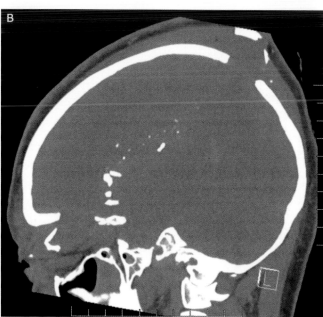

FIGURE 7–3. **(A)** MPR parasagittal image from helical axial data. Brain (soft) tissue window setting shows projectile track, entering left orbit and exiting the left posterior parietal bone. **(B)** Same image as in A. Bone window setting.

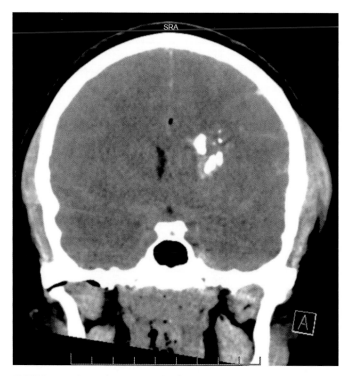

FIGURE 7–2. Coronal MPR. Note that fresh blood is seen in the left lateral ventricle.

occipital bone to the vertex of the skull. The lens of the eyes will be exposed to radiation. In this example of risks versus benefits, the risks of the radiation exposure are not as great as the benefits of performing the procedure in this manner.

8

Paranasal Sinuses

INDICATIONS

Most commonly used to evaluate for an inflammatory condition or a neoplasm and to follow up on inflammatory disease during treatment.

IMAGING APPLICATIONS

Patient/Part Positioning

Position the patient either supine or prone. If prone, position the patient with their chin extended and the mental point resting on the table. Position the patient's head so the midsagittal plane is vertical and centered to the table. The interpupillary line should be level without any rotation or tilt. See Chapter 4.

Breathing Instructions

Quiet breathing.

Scan Range

From just beneath the maxilla through the entire frontal sinus area. See Figures 8-1 to 8-4.

Gantry Angulation

From the lateral scout view, tilt the gantry to be perpendicular to the hard palate.

Field of View

Small, 12 to 15 cm.

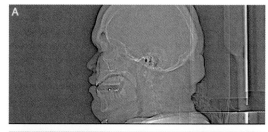
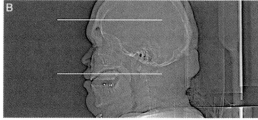

FIGURE 8–1. Lateral scout **(A)** with slice overlay **(B)** showing scan range from just beneath the maxilla superiorly through the entire frontal sinus area. Note that the length of the slice overlay lines indicates the size of the field of view.

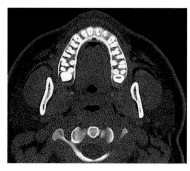

FIGURE 8–2. Axial bone window of initial slice. Note the good symmetrical positioning.

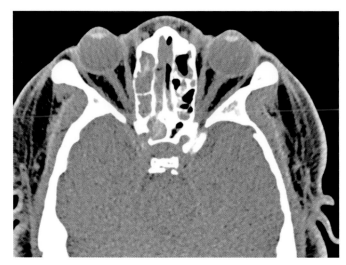

FIGURE 8–3. Axial soft tissue window at the level of the orbits. Note the lens of the eyes.

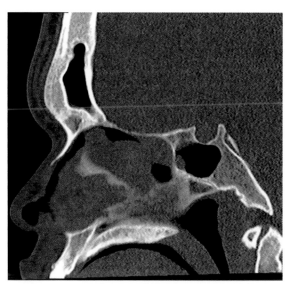

FIGURE 8–6. Sagittal MPR bone window showing opacification of the ethmoid and sphenoid sinuses on this image.

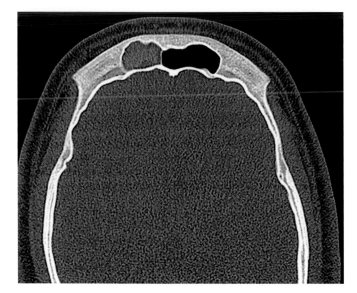

FIGURE 8–4. Axial bone window showing frontal sinus with opacification of the right frontal sinus area.

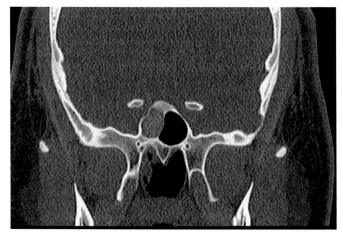

FIGURE 8–5. Coronal MPR bone window image showing opacification of the sphenoid sinus.

Slice Thickness

Reconstructed slice thickness of 3 mm or less for better spatial resolution.

Table Movement

Caudocranial.

Reconstruction Kernel/Algorithm

Soft tissue and bone algorithms should be used.

Window Level (WL)/Window Width (WW)

Approximate setting for:

- Bone window: +450 HU = WL; +1500 HU = WW
- Soft tissue: +50 HU = WL; +350 HU = WW

SPECIAL CONSIDERATIONS

Multiplanar Reconstruction (MPR)

Using an axial image, position the slice overlay to produce coronal MPR images (Figure 8–5) and position it vertical to produce sagittal MPR images (Figure 8–6).

Contrast Media

Usually, no intravenous contrast is needed unless a neoplasm is seen. Contrast should be directed by a radiologist.

Radiation Reduction Option

Helical mode may result in less radiation when compared to axial mode when considering coronal and sagittal MPRs.

Reference

International Atomic Energy Agency (IAEA). Radiation protection of patients with cataract. Accessed March 2022. https://www.iaea.org/resources/rpop/health-professionals/radiology/cataract/patients.

9
Maxillofacial Bones

INDICATIONS

Most commonly used to evaluate for trauma or tumor.

IMAGING APPLICATIONS

Patient/Part Positioning

Position the patient supine and headfirst into the gantry. Position the patient's head so there is no rotation and the midsagittal plane is straight and centered to the table. Adjust the interpupillary line to be straight with no tilt. Adjust the head so the orbitomeatal line (OML) is perpendicular to the table. See Chapter 4.

Breathing Instructions

Suspend breathing during the scan.

Scan Range

Scan from the superior orbital margin down through the mental point of the mandible. See Figures 9-1 to 9-4.

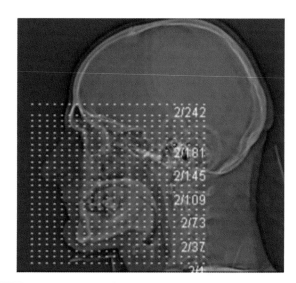

FIGURE 9-2. Lateral scout of the head with axial slice overlay for maxillofacial bone examination. Note that the slice overlay also provides information regarding the FOV for anatomic coverage.

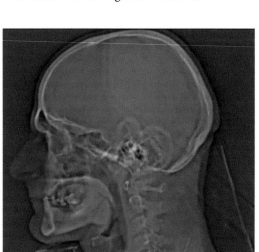

FIGURE 9-1. Lateral scout of the head.

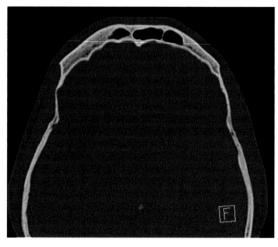

FIGURE 9-3. Axial image showing the initial slice level. The frontal sinus is also shown. This is a bone window.

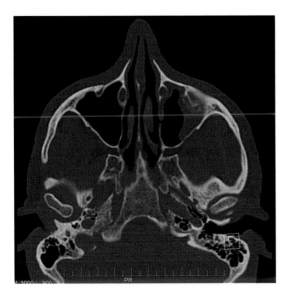

FIGURE 9–4. Axial image at the level of the maxillary sinuses. Note the symmetry of the anatomy. This indicates very little rotation and allows for better comparison between left- and right-sided structures.

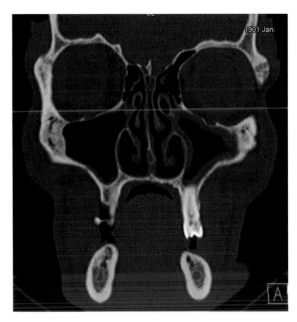

FIGURE 9–5. Coronal MPR showing the orbital, ethmoid, and maxillary bony structures.

Gantry Angulation

With the gantry angulation at 0 degrees, adjust the patient's head so the OML is vertical.

Field of View

Small, 12 to 15 cm.

Slice Thickness

Use reconstructed slice thickness of 3 mm or less for better spatial resolution. Thin-section coronal multiplanar reconstruction (MPR) images are also helpful.

Table Movement

Craniocaudal.

Reconstruction Kernel/Algorithm

Soft tissue and bone algorithms.

Window Level (WL)/Window Width (WW)

Approximate setting for:

- Brain tissue: +40 HU = WL; +100 HU = WW
- Bone window: +300 HU = WL; +1500 HU = WW

SPECIAL CONSIDERATIONS

Multiplanar Reconstruction

Using an axial image, position the slice overlay to produce coronal MPR images (Figure 9–5) and position vertical to produce sagittal MPR images (Figure 9–6). Extend the slice overlay to cover the entire region.

Contrast Media

Usually no contrast media is needed.

Radiation Reduction Option

Position orbital shielding anterior to the orbits to reduce direct radiation exposure.

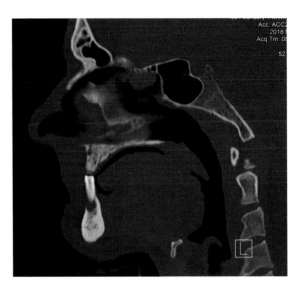

FIGURE 9–6. Sagittal MPR very near the midline. Note the saddle-shaped sella turcica, the sphenoid sinus, and the clivus.

10
Orbits

INDICATIONS

Most commonly used to evaluate for trauma, tumor, or foreign body.

IMAGING APPLICATIONS

Patient/Part Positioning

Position the patient supine and headfirst into the gantry. Position the patient's head so the midsagittal plane is straight and the interpupillary line is perpendicular to the midsagittal plane. Adjust the head so the orbitomeatal line (OML) is perpendicular to the table. See Chapter 4.

Breathing Instructions

Suspend breathing during the scan.

Scan Range

Scan from the superior orbital margin down through the inferior orbital margin. See Figures 10–1 to 10–3.

Gantry Angulation

With the gantry angulation at 0 degrees, adjust the patient's head so the OML is vertical.

Field of View

Small, 12 to 15 cm.

Slice Thickness

Use reconstructed slice thickness of 3 mm or less for better spatial resolution. Thin-section coronal multiplanar reconstruction (MPR) images are also helpful. Thin-section sagittal oblique MPR images are very helpful when aligned along the optic nerve.

Table Movement

Craniocaudal.

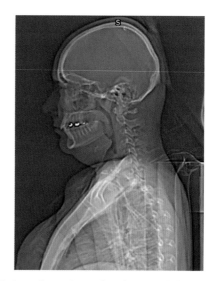

FIGURE 10–1. Lateral scout image for orbits provided with this exam. Question: Do you see anything wrong with this scout? The scan range has been extended, allowing for unnecessary radiation exposure.

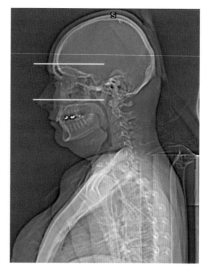

FIGURE 10–2. Lateral scout with axial slice overlay for orbits.

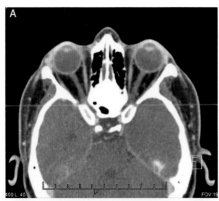

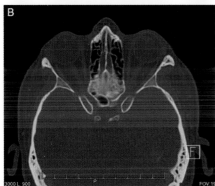

FIGURE 10–3. Axial soft tissue **(A)** window of the orbits showing good view of the globe, optic nerve, medial and lateral rectus muscles, and retro-orbital fat. Good position with no rotation or tilt. Bone window **(B)** allows for good evaluation of bony structures.

Reconstruction Kernel/Algorithm

Soft tissue and bone algorithms.

Window Level (WL)/Window Width (WW)

Approximate setting for:

- Soft tissue: +40 HU = WL; +400 HU = WW
- Bone window: +300 HU = WL; +1500 HU = WW

SPECIAL CONSIDERATIONS

- MPR: Using an axial image, position the slice overlay to produce coronal MPR images (Figure 10–4) and position vertical to produce sagittal MPR images (Figure 10–5). Extend the slice overlay to cover the entire area of interest.
- Figure 10–6 shows a hemangioma from a different patient. The coronal and sagittal MPR images help to show the displacement of the optic nerve for treatment planning.

Contrast Media

Use intravenous (IV) contrast when tumor is suspected.

Radiation Reduction Option

Position orbital shielding anterior to the orbits to reduce direct radiation exposure.

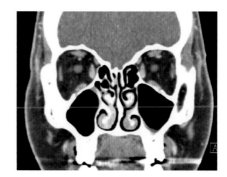

FIGURE 10–4. Coronal MPR showing good view of orbital anatomy. The 4 main rectus muscles are positioned like the face of a clock. The superior rectus muscle is at 12 o'clock, and the inferior rectus muscle is at 6 o'clock. The medial rectus muscle and the lateral rectus muscle are in the 3 o'clock or 9 o'clock position depending on which orbit is being viewed. Hypodense fat is seen surrounding the optic nerve. Note the metallic streak artifact.

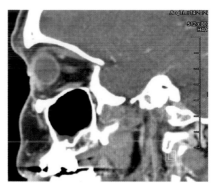

FIGURE 10–5. Sagittal oblique MPR along the long axis of the optic nerve, showing the superior and inferior rectus muscles, globe of the eye, and optic nerve with hypodense retro-orbital fat. Note the metallic streak artifact from dental work.

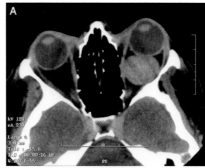

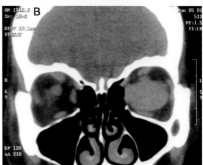

FIGURE 10–6. Axial **(A)** and coronal MPR **(B)** of a retro-orbital hemangioma. These images are from 2001 and show the diagnostic quality of the technology at that time. (Panel A: Reprinted from Grey ML, Alinani JM. *CT and MRI Pathology: A Pocket Atlas*. McGraw-Hill; 2018, with permission from The McGraw-Hill Companies.)

11

Temporal Bone: Interior Auditory Canal (IAC)

INDICATIONS

Hearing loss, chronic ear infection, neoplasms, otomastoid inflammatory disease, suspected disease of the inner ear, pre-surgery evaluation, postsurgery evaluation, radiation therapy treatment planning, congenital anomalies, and trauma.

IMAGING APPLICATIONS

Patient/Part Positioning

Position the patient supine and headfirst into the gantry. Position the patient's head so the midsagittal plane is straight and the interpupillary line is straight. Adjust the head so the orbito-meatal line is perpendicular to the table. See Chapter 4.

Breathing Instructions

Suspend breathing.

Scan Range

For axial images, scan from the most superior portion of the mastoid air cells through to the stylomastoid foramen inferiorly. See Figures 11–1 to 11–3.

Gantry Angulation

With the gantry angulation at 0 degrees, adjust the patient's head so the OML is vertical.

Field of View

Use a small field of view (≤12 cm) for better spatial resolution.

Slice Thickness

Reconstructed slice thickness should not exceed 1.5 mm.

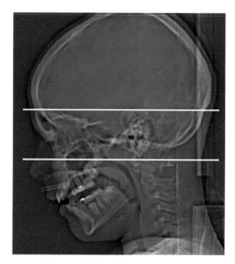

FIGURE 11–1. Lateral scout image with axial slice overlay indicating scan range.

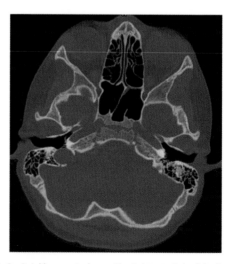

FIGURE 11–2. Axial bone window with slight rotation of the head at the level of the mastoid air cells.

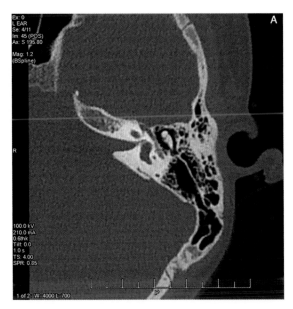 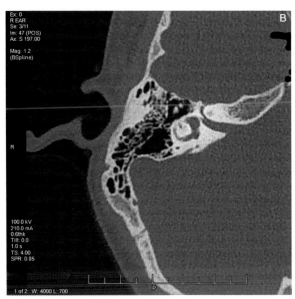

FIGURE 11–3. Axial bone window magnified images of the left **(A)** and right **(B)** temporal bone region.

Table Movement

Craniocaudal.

Reconstruction Kernel/Algorithm

Soft tissue and bone high-resolution algorithms.

Window Level (WL)/Window Width (WW)

Approximate setting for:

- Bone window: +700 HU = WL; +4000 HU = WW

SPECIAL CONSIDERATIONS

Multiplanar Reconstruction (MPR)

For coronal oblique images, align slice overlay perpendicular to the semicircular canal (SCC). This may be referred to as the Stenvers plane (Figure 11–4).

For sagittal oblique images, align the slice overlay parallel to the SCC. This may be referred to as the Pöschl plane (Figure 11–5).

Contrast Media

Intravenous contrast media may be used to evaluate vascular pathology (eg, tumors and certain types of infections).

Radiation Reduction Option

Angle the gantry to avoid the lens of the eyes. Align the gantry parallel with the supraorbital meatal line (SOML).

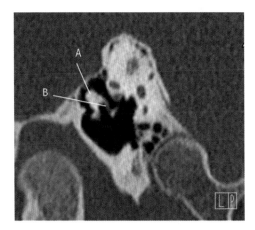

FIGURE 11–5. Sagittal MPR bone window showing the malleus (A) and incus (B) ossicles within the middle ear.

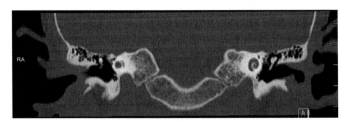

FIGURE 11–4. Bilateral coronal MPR bone windowing showing the cochlea.

12
Soft Tissue Neck

INDICATIONS

Tumors, infections, congenital disorders, vascular lesions, trauma, and posttreatment (surgical and radiation therapy) evaluation.

IMAGING APPLICATIONS

Patient/Part Positioning

Position the patient supine and straight on the patient couch. Center the patient's body and neck to be in the center of the patient couch and headfirst in the gantry. Instruct the patient to lower their shoulders to reduce beam hardening. See Chapter 4.

Instruct the patient to breathe quietly, suppress swallowing, and avoid coughing.

- To better visualize the laryngeal ventricle, instruct the patient to use an [i] phonation.
- To better visualize the pyriform sinuses and postcricoid region, instruct the patient to use the modified Valsalva maneuver.

Scan Range

From the superior orbital rim to the apex of the lungs. See Figure 12–1.

Gantry Angulation

Using the lateral scout image, adjust the slice alignment tool angulation to be perpendicular to the major portion of the neck. Angle the slice overlay in a manner to avoid imaging dental implants and large amounts of dental amalgam because they

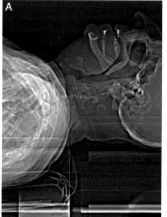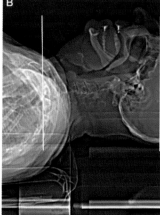

FIGURE 12–1. (A) A lateral scout image of the neck. **(B)** In this image, lines are placed superiorly at the level of the superior orbital rim and inferiorly at the level of the apex of the lungs to acquire axial images.

may produce image artifacts and be detrimental to the quality of the image. If necessary, use separate angulation to avoid x-ray interactions and improve image quality.

Slice Thickness

Contiguous axial 5-mm slice thickness may be adequate. However, if better image detail is needed, a 2- to 3-mm slice thickness can be used.

Table Movement

Scan from cranial to caudal to reduce beam hardening artifact at the level of the thoracic inlet caused by intravenous (IV) contrast.

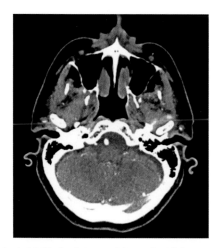

FIGURE 12–2. Axial CT of soft tissue of the neck with IV contrast. Note the contrast-enhanced basilar artery located along the midline and at the level of the lower pons.

Reconstruction Kernel/Algorithm

Soft tissue kernel (Figure 12–2). If there is pathology involving the bone or cartilage, reconstruct the raw data with a high-resolution bone algorithm.

Window Level (WL)/Window Width (WW)

Approximate setting for:

- Soft tissue: +50 HU = WL; +250 to +350 HU = WW

SPECIAL CONSIDERATIONS

Multiplanar Reconstruction (MPR)

Using an axial image, position the slice overlay to produce coronal MPR images (Figure 12–3B) and position vertical to produce sagittal MPR images (Figure 12–3A). For the sagittal image, use an odd number of slices and align the middle slice along the midline to produce a midline sagittal image of the throat region.

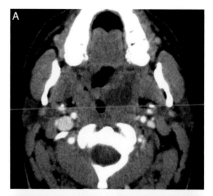

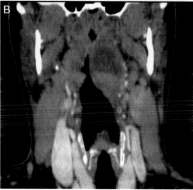

FIGURE 12–4. Peritonsillar abscess. Axial **(A)** and coronal **(B)** contrast-enhanced CT images show low attenuation with minimal rim enhancement in left tonsillar region representing phlegmon or early abscess of the faucial tonsil. (Reprinted from Grey ML, Alinani JM. *CT and MRI Pathology: A Pocket Atlas.* McGraw-Hill; 2018, with permission from The McGraw-Hill Companies.)

Contrast Media

Use an IV contrast bolus of 80 to 100 mL administrated at 1 to 2 mL/s with a delay of 80 to 100 seconds prior to image acquisition. After the IV contrast has been administered, follow with a rapid saline drip at the same rate to allow the contrast media in the IV line to enter into the patient. (See Figure 12–4A and 4B.)

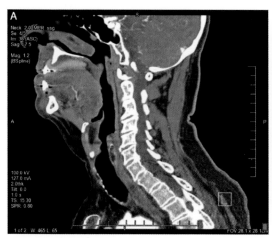

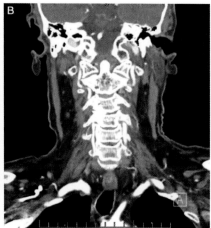

FIGURE 12–3. **(A)** A parasagittal MPR just slightly off the midline. **(B)** A coronal MPR. Note the vertebral arteries with IV contrast and the second cervical (C2) vertebra.

13

CT Angiography (CTA) Neck: Carotids

INDICATIONS

CT angiography (CTA) of the neck is used to evaluate the carotid and vertebral arteries from the aortic arch to the circle of Willis and to detect occlusion and thrombosis, carotid artery stenosis, aneurysms, vascular malformations, or ongoing bleeding.

IMAGING APPLICATIONS

Patient/Part Positioning

Position the patient supine and headfirst in the gantry with their arms by their side. Position the head straight on the table with the orbitomeatal line perpendicular to the table. Align the midsagittal plane of the patient's head so there is no rotation. Adjust the interpupillary line so it is perpendicular to the midline sagittal plane of the patient's head (Figures 13–1). See Chapter 4.

Breathing Instructions

Suspend respiration.

Scan Range

Caudocranial from the aortic arch (mid-chest) to the vertex. See Figures 13–2, 13–3, and 13–4.

Gantry Angulation

Gantry angulation is 0 degrees.

Slice Thickness

Thin-section images for increased spatial resolution.

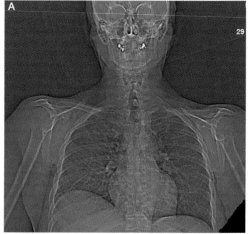

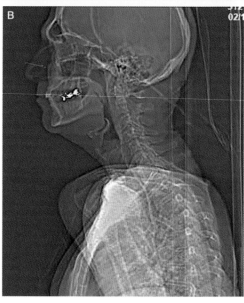

FIGURE 13–1. (A and B) AP scout (**A**) and lateral scout (**B**) images.

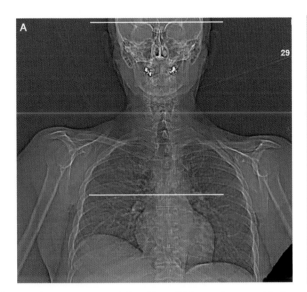
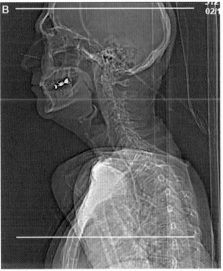

FIGURE 13-2. (A and B) Anteroposterior **(A)** and lateral **(B)** scout images with slice overlay indicating the scan range and field of view.

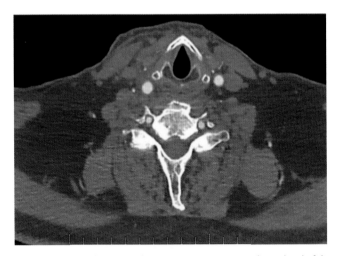

FIGURE 13-3. Axial image with intravenous contrast at a lower level of the neck. This is a different patient from the other images. Note the common carotid arteries medial of the jugular veins and the vertebral arteries.

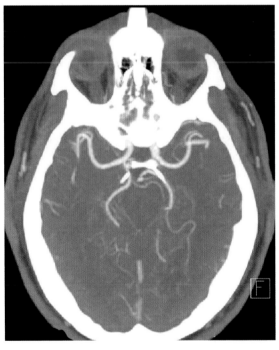

FIGURE 13-4. Axial image of the circle of Willis at the superior level of the scan range.

Table Movement

Scan from caudal to cranial to follow the flow of the contrast agent in the vascular structures.

Reconstruction Kernel/Algorithm

Soft tissue algorithm.

Window Level (WL)/Window Width (WW)

Approximate setting for:

- Soft tissue window: +80 HU = WL; +700 HU = WW

SPECIAL CONSIDERATIONS

- Bolus triggering region of interest (ROI) may be placed in the carotid artery.
- Multiplanar reconstruction (MPR): Using an axial image, position the slice overlay to produce coronal MPR images and position vertical to produce sagittal MPR images (Figure 13–5).
- Curved MPR of the entire path of the vessel may be helpful.
- Minimum intensity projection (MIP). See Figure 13–3.
- Shaded surface display volume rendering may be helpful. See Figures 13–6A and 13–6B.

Contrast Media

Use an intravenous injection of 50 to 75 mL of nonionic iodinated contrast with a saline chaser at 4 to 5 mL/s injection rate. Use the descending aorta to place the ROI for bolus triggering with a threshold of 100 HU. See Figure 13–7.

Radiation Reduction Option

CTA of the neck provides less radiation exposure as compared to catheter angiography.

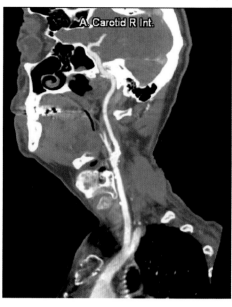

FIGURE 13–5. Sagittal MIP of the right internal carotid artery. Note the bifurcation of the common carotid artery.

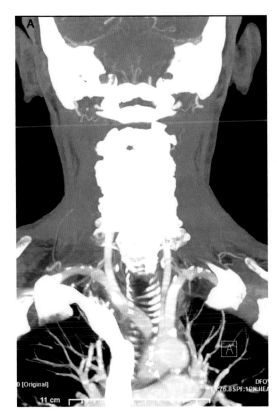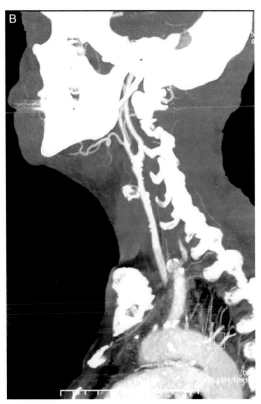

FIGURE 13-6. Coronal **(A)** and sagittal **(B)** MIP images.

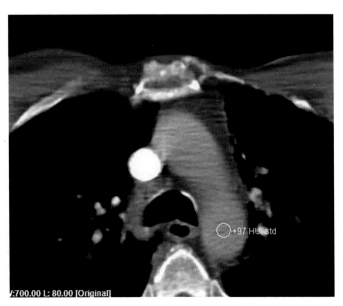

FIGURE 13-7. Axial monitoring image used for bolus triggering. The ROI is positioned in the descending portion of the aortic arch.

14
Cervical Spine

INDICATIONS

Trauma, degenerative conditions, postoperative evaluation, infection, neoplastic conditions, inflammatory conditions, and congenital or developmental abnormalities.

IMAGING APPLICATIONS

Patient/Part Positioning

Position the patient supine and headfirst in the gantry. Adjust the patient so they are straight and centered on the table with no rotation. See Chapter 4.

Scan Range

The entire cervical spine external auditory meatus (EAM) through T1 vertebra. See Figures 14–1 and 14–2.

Gantry Angulation

Angle the gantry to be parallel to the intervertebral disk.

Field of View

Small field of view, 12 to 15 cm. See Figure 14– 3.

Slice Thickness

Reconstructed slice thickness of 3 mm or less for better spatial resolution.

Table Movement

Craniocaudal.

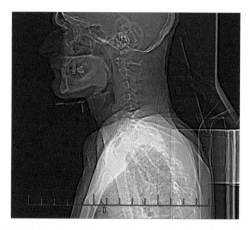

FIGURE 14–1. Lateral scout for cervical spine. Note that the patient's arms are down by their side with shoulders pulled down.

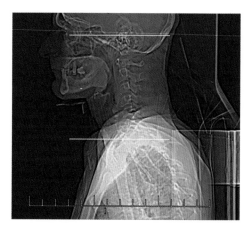

FIGURE 14–2. Lateral scout of cervical spine with slice overlay. Scan range is from approximately the level of the EAM through the T1 vertebra.

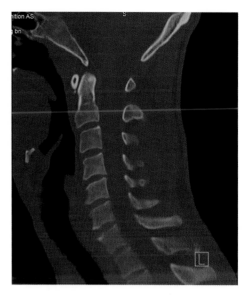

FIGURE 14–3. Axial bone window at the level of C1 (atlas). The odontoid process (dens) of C2 (axis) and the transverse foramen are also clearly seen.

Reconstruction Kernel/Algorithm

Soft tissue and bone algorithms should be used.

Window Level (WL)/Window Width (WW)

Approximate setting for:

- Bone window: +900 HU = WL; +3000 HU = WW
- Tissue window: +40-50 HU = WL; +350-400 HU = WW

SPECIAL CONSIDERATIONS

Multiplanar Reconstruction (MPR)

Using an axial image, position the slice overlay to produce coronal MPR images (Figure 14–4) and position vertical to produce sagittal MPR images (Figure 14–5). For the sagittal MPR, use

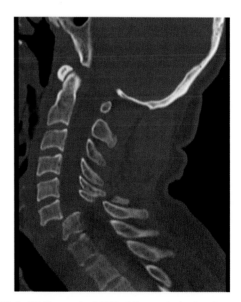

FIGURE 14–5. Sagittal MPR of the cervical spine.

an odd number of slices in the slice overlay so the middle image will be along the midline. Extend the slice overlay to cover the all vertebrae. This will allow the intervertebral foramen and the spinal nerve roots to be visualized.

Figure 14–6 is a midline sagittal MPR showing a type 4 spondylolisthesis in a different patient.

Contrast Media

Usually, no intravenous contrast is needed.

Radiation Reduction Options

- Use automatic tube current modulation.
- Use iterative reconstruction technique.

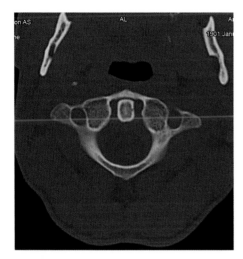

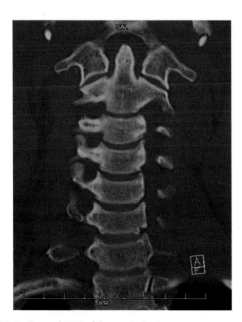

FIGURE 14–4. Coronal MPR of the cervical spine.

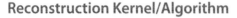

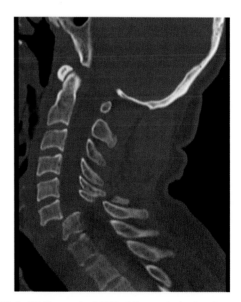

FIGURE 14–6. Midline sagittal MPR of the cervical spine. Bone window shows a type 4 spondylolisthesis at the level of C6/C7. (Reprinted from Grey ML, Alinani JM. *CT and MRI Pathology: A Pocket Atlas*. McGraw-Hill; 2018, with permission from The McGraw-Hill Companies.)

15
Thoracic Spine

INDICATIONS

Trauma, degenerative conditions, postoperative evaluation, infection, neoplastic conditions, inflammatory conditions, and congenital or developmental abnormalities.

IMAGING APPLICATIONS

Patient/Part Positioning

Position the patient supine and headfirst in the gantry. Adjust the patient so they are straight and centered on the table with no rotation. Position the patient's arms out of the imaging field. See Chapter 4.

Scan Range

The entire thoracic spine, C7 through L1 vertebrae. See Figures 15–1 to 15–3.

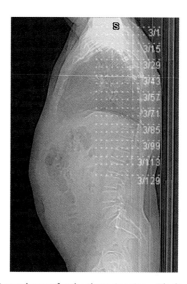

FIGURE 15–2. Lateral scout for the thoracic spine with slice overlay. The field of view is indicated by the length of the lines. Note that the slice overlay extends further than necessary (L2-L3) into the disk space.

Gantry Angulation

Angle the gantry to be parallel to the intervertebral disk. However, the exam may be performed in spiral mode. Images shown in Figures 15–2 through 15–5 were scanned in spiral mode. Gantry angulation for spiral mode is 0 degrees.

Field of View

Small, 12 to 15 cm.

Slice Thickness

Reconstructed slice thickness of 3 mm or less for better spatial resolution.

Table Movement

Craniocaudal.

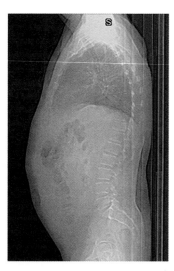

FIGURE 15–1. Lateral scout for thoracic spine. Patient's arms are positioned above their head.

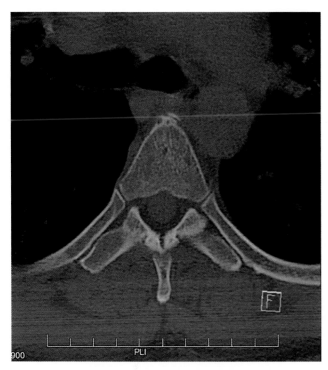

FIGURE 15–3. Axial bone window of the thoracic spine at the level of the carina (T4/T5).

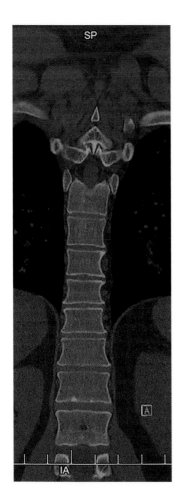

FIGURE 15–4. Coronal MPR of the thoracic spine. Note the straight positioning of the spine. This helps when reconstructing the sagittal MPR images. Also seen are the costocardiac angles of the lungs.

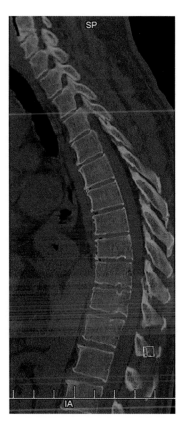

FIGURE 15–5. Sagittal MPR of the thoracic spine along the midline. Midline sagittal is helpful in evaluating for alignment of the vertebrae and spinal canal.

Reconstruction Kernel/Algorithm

Soft tissue and bone algorithms should be used.

Window Level (WL)/Window Width (WW)

Approximate setting for:

- Bone window: +900 HU = WL; +3000 HU = WW
- Tissue window: +40-50 HU = WL; +350-400 HU = WW

SPECIAL CONSIDERATIONS

Multiplanar Reconstruction (MPR)

Using an axial image, position the slice overlay to produce coronal MPR images (Figure 15–4) and position vertically to produce sagittal MPR images (Figure 15–5). For the sagittal MPR, use an odd number of slices in the slice overlay so the middle image will be along the midline. Extend the slice overlay to cover the entire vertebra. This will allow the intervertebral foramen and the spinal nerve roots to be visualized.

Contrast Media

Usually, no intravenous contrast is needed.

Radiation Reduction Options

- Use automatic tube current modulation.
- Use iterative reconstruction technique.

16
Lumbar Spine

INDICATIONS

Trauma, degenerative conditions, postoperative evaluation, infection, neoplastic conditions, inflammatory conditions, and congenital or developmental abnormalities.

IMAGING APPLICATIONS

Patient/Part Positioning

Position the patient supine and headfirst in the gantry. Adjust the patient so they are straight and centered on the table with no rotation. Position the patient's arms out of the imaging field. See Chapter 4.

Scan Range

The entire lumbar spine from T12 through S1.

Gantry Angulation

Angle the gantry to be parallel to the intervertebral disk. When the exam calls for the entire lumbar spine to be scanned, the gantry angulation is set at 0 degrees and helical mode is used. See Figures 16–1 and 16–2.

Field of View

Small, 12 to 15 cm.

Slice Thickness

Reconstructed slice thickness of 3 mm or less for better spatial resolution.

Table Movement

Craniocaudal.

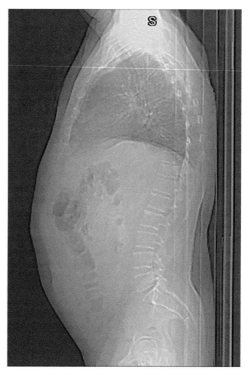

FIGURE 16–1. Lateral scout for lumbar spine. Note that this scout was used for multiple exams on this patient.

Reconstruction Kernel/Algorithm

Soft tissue and bone algorithms.

Window Level (WL)/Window Width (WW)

Approximate setting for:

- Bone window: +900 HU = WL; +3000 HU = WW
- Tissue window: +40-50 HU = WL; +350-400 HU = WW

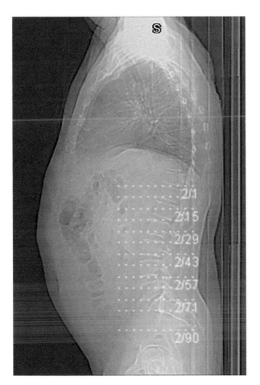

FIGURE 16–2. Lateral scout for lumbar spine with slice overlay.

SPECIAL CONSIDERATIONS

Multiplanar Reconstruction (MPR)

Using an axial image, position the slice overlay vertically to produce sagittal MPR images (Figures 16–3 and 16–4). For the sagittal MPR, use an odd number of slices in the slice overlay so the middle image will be along the midline. Extend the slice overlay to cover the entire vertebrae. This will allow the intervertebral foramen and the spinal nerve roots to be visualized.

Figure 16–5 shows a burst fracture in a different patient.

Contrast Media

Usually, no intravenous contrast is needed.

Radiation Reduction Options

- Use automatic tube current modulation.
- Use iterative reconstruction technique.

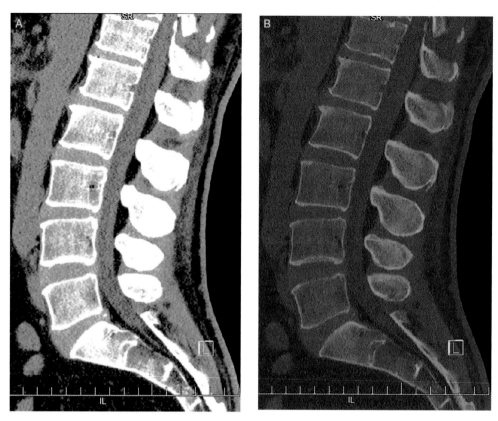

FIGURE 16–3. Midline sagittal MPR of the lumbar spine **(A)** with soft tissue window and **(B)** with bone window. Note the good alignment of the vertebral bodies.

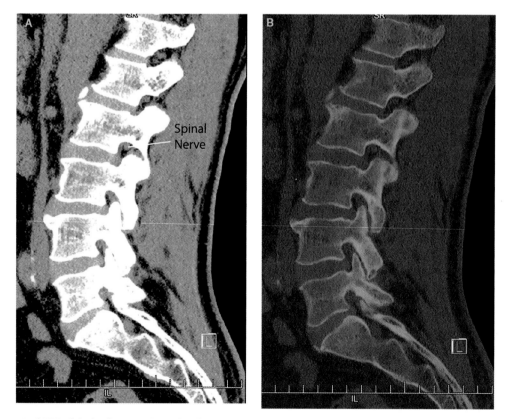

FIGURE 16–4. Parasagittal MPR of the lumbar spine **(A)** with soft tissue window and **(B)** with bone window. Note the spinal nerve **(A)** exiting the spinal cord through the intervertebral foramen. Good view of the facet joint **(B)** at L3/L4 showing the inferior articular process of L3 and the superior articular process of L4.

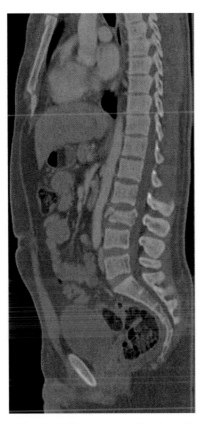

FIGURE 16–5. Burst fracture at L3. (Reprinted from Grey ML, Alinani JM. *CT and MRI Pathology: A Pocket Atlas*. McGraw-Hill; 2018, with permission from The McGraw-Hill Companies.)

17

Chest, Abdomen, and Pelvis (CAP)

INDICATIONS

See Chapters 18 and 22.

IMAGING APPLICATIONS

The chest, abdomen, and pelvis (CAP) exam may be performed as 2 separate exams following the scout views (see Figures 17–3A and 17–3B). Figures 17–4 and 17–5 are from a different patient than Figures 17–1, 17–3A, and 17–3B.

Patient/Part Positioning

Position the patient supine and headfirst in the gantry. Adjust the patient so they are straight and flat (no rotation of the body) on the table. After an intravenous (IV) is in place, position the patient's arms above their head. If needed, support the patient's arms on a pillow above their head. This is to be performed prior to acquiring the anteroposterior (AP) and lateral scout images (Figures 17–1 and 17–2).

Breathing Instructions

Full inhalation for the chest exam. Exhalation for the abdomen and pelvis exam.

Scan Range

See specific instructions regarding the scan range for each exam from the routine chest (Figures 17–3A and 17–4) and routine abdomen and pelvis (Figures 17–3B and 17–5) exams.

Gantry Angulation

Gantry angulation is 0 degrees.

Field of View (FOV)

For the chest exam, the FOV should be large enough to include the patient's chest region. For the abdomen and pelvis exam, the FOV should be large enough to include the patient's body.

Slick Thickness

Reconstructed slice thickness of 5 to 8 mm is commonly used. A slice thickness of 3 mm or less provides better spatial resolution.

Table Movement

Craniocaudal. Perform the chest exam before the abdomen and pelvis exam for better IV contrast visibility of the pulmonary hilar region.

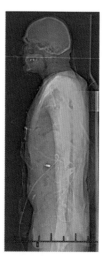

FIGURES 17–1. Lateral scout image. Note that this is a trauma patient who is unable to raise their arms above their head.

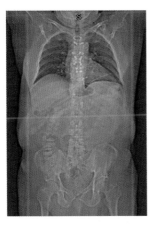

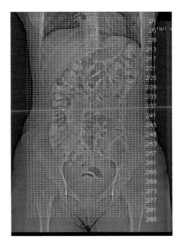

FIGURES 17–5. AP scout with slice overlay showing the scan range for a routine abdomen and pelvis exam. Note that Figure 17–5 is from a different patient than in Figures 17–1, 17–2, 17–3A, and 17–3B.

Reconstruction Kernel/Algorithm

Soft tissue and lung algorithms should be used. Bone window may be helpful in trauma cases.

Window Level (WL)/Window Width (WW)

Approximate setting for:

- Soft tissue window: +40 HU = WL; +400 HU = WW
- Lung window: –200 HU = WL; +2000 HU = WW
- Bone window: +300 HU = WL; +1500 HU = WW

SPECIAL CONSIDERATIONS

- Multiplanar Reconstruction (MPR)
  - Coronal MPR to the body axis.
  - Sagittal MPR to the body axis.
- Place bolus triggering in the ascending aorta if using IV contrast.

Contrast Media

IV contrast exams may vary depending on the purpose of the exam. For routine purposes, an injection rate of 2 mL/s with a total volume of 150 mL is sufficient. However, for vascular purposes, higher injection rates of 3 to 4 mL/s are suggested. A large-bore IV catheter (eg, 18-gauge) placed in a large antecubital vein is recommended. A saline bolus is used to flush remaining contrast from the IV line into the patient. Bolus triggering (bolus tracking) (region of interest) is placed in the ascending aorta. Scan delay is set before actual data acquisition begins.

Radiation Reduction Options

- Use automatic tube modulation with patient's arms raised above their head. If IV contrast is being used, place the IV prior to positioning.
- Use iterative reconstruction technique.

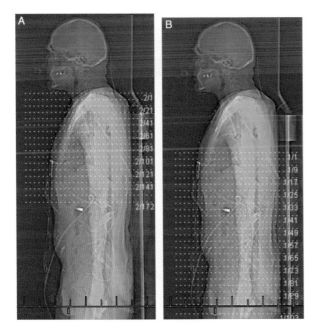

FIGURES 17–2. AP scout of a different patient than in Figure 17–1. The patient's arms are positioned above their head.

FIGURES 17–3. Same trauma patient as in Figure 17–1. Slice overlays for lateral chest **(A)** and abdomen and pelvis **(B)** are shown. There should be overlapping of the anatomy where the 2 exams meet.

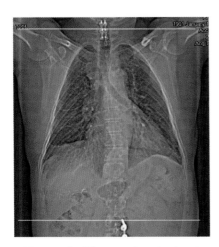

FIGURES 17–4. AP scout of a different patient showing the scan range for a routine chest exam. Note that Figure 17–4 is from a different patient than in Figures 17–1, 17–2, 17–3A, and 17–3B.

18

Routine Chest

INDICATIONS

Staging and follow-up of lung cancer; evaluation of cardiothoracic disease, cardiovascular abnormalities, pulmonary emboli, blunt and penetrating trauma, and pulmonary disease; CT-guided interventional procedures; and radiation therapy treatment planning.

IMAGING APPLICATIONS

Patient/Part Positioning

Position the patient supine and headfirst in the gantry. Adjust the patient so they are straight and flat (no rotation of the body) on the table. After an intravenous (IV) is in place, position the patient's arms above their head. If needed, support the patient's arms on a pillow above their head. This is to be performed prior to acquiring the anteroposterior (AP) Figure 18-1A.

Breathing Instructions

Full inhalation. If the patient has dyspnea and is unable to hold their breath during the scan, swallow breathing may be helpful.

Scan Range

Use AP (Figure 18–1B) and lateral scouts to assist with the placement of the slice overlay for axial images. Extend the slice overlay from the thoracic inlet (located just above the apex of the lung) inferiorly to include the adrenal glands. See Figures 18–2 and 18–3.

Gantry Angulation

Gantry angulation is 0 degrees.

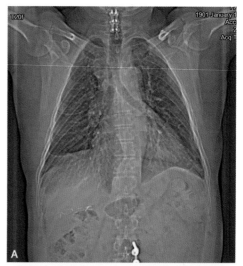

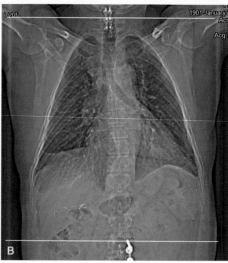

FIGURE 18–1. **(A)** AP scout of the chest. **(B)** AP scout of the chest with slice overlay showing the scan range and axial slice orientation indicated by the superiorly and inferiorly placed lines.

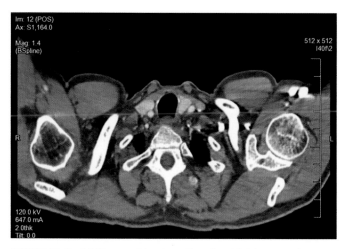

FIGURE 18–2. Axial image of the chest. Note that this is image 12 (upper left-hand corner) of the data set.

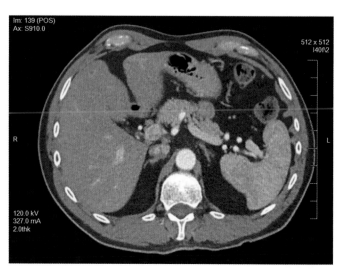

FIGURE 18–3. Axial image of the chest at the level of the adrenal glands. Good image detail is due to the 2.0-mm slice thickness. Note that this is image 139 (upper left-hand corner) of the data set.

Field of View

The field of view should be large enough to include the patient's chest region.

Slice Thickness

Reconstructed slice thickness of 5 to 8 mm is commonly used.

Table Movement

Craniocaudal. If performing a combined exam of the chest, abdomen, and pelvis, imaging of the chest is performed prior to the abdomen and pelvis for better IV contrast visibility of the pulmonary hilar region.

Reconstruction Kernel/Algorithm

Soft tissue and lung algorithms. Bone window may be helpful in trauma cases.

Window Level (WL)/Window Width (WW)

Approximate setting for:

- Soft tissue window: +40 HU = WL; +400 HU = WW
- Lung window: –200 HU = WL; +2000 HU = WW
- Bone window; +300 HU = WL; +1500 HU = WW

SPECIAL CONSIDERATIONS

- Multiplanar reconstruction (MPR)
  - Coronal MPR to the body axis.
  - Sagittal MPR to the body axis.
- Place bolus triggering in the ascending aorta if using IV contrast.

Contrast Media

If needed, IV contrast exams may vary depending on the purpose of the exam. For routine purposes, an injection rate of 2 mL/s with a total volume of 150 mL is sufficient. However, for vascular purposes, higher injection rates of 3 to 4 mL/s are suggested. A large-bore IV catheter (eg, 18 gauge) placed in a large antecubital vein is recommended. A saline bolus is used to flush the remaining contrast from the IV line into the patient. Bolus triggering (region of interest) is placed in the ascending aorta. Scan delay is set before actual data acquisition begins.

Radiation Reduction Options

- Use automatic tube modulation.
- Use iterative reconstruction technique.

19

High-Resolution Chest

INDICATIONS

Evaluation of diffuse pulmonary diseases such as chronic obstructive pulmonary disease (COPD) and emphysema.

IMAGING APPLICATIONS

Patient/Part Positioning

Position the patient supine and headfirst in the gantry. Adjust the patient so they are straight and flat (no rotation of the body) on the table. Position the patient's arms above their head (Figure 19–1A).

When fibrosis is suspected, position the patient prone.

Breathing Instructions

Suspend inspiration. Suspended expiration is helpful to evaluate for trapped air.

Scan Range

Use anteroposterior (AP) and lateral scouts to assist with the placement of the slice overlay for axial images. Extend the slice overlay from the thoracic outlet (located just above the apex of the lung) through the lung to the level of the adrenal glands (Figure 19–1B).

Gantry Angulation

No gantry angle is needed.

Field of View

The field of view should be large enough to include the patient's chest region.

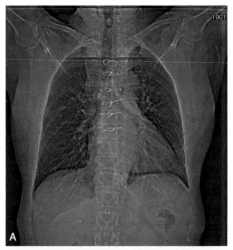

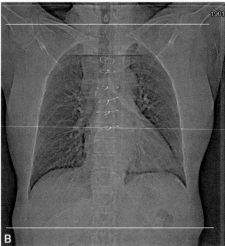

FIGURE 19–1. **(A)** AP scout of the chest. **(B)** AP scout of the chest with slice overlay showing the scan range and axial slice orientation indicated by the superiorly and inferiorly placed lines.

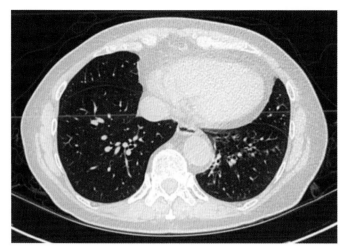

FIGURE 19-2. Lung window.

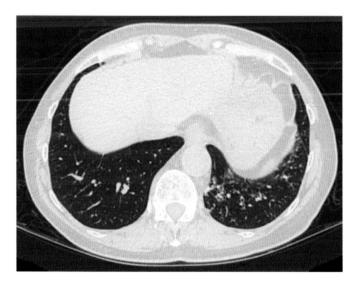

FIGURE 19-3. Same patient as shown in Figure 19-2. Axial lung window image showing bronchiectasis of the left lower lobe.

Slice Thickness

Thin-section (1-2 mm) imaging with a 10- to 20-mm gap between slices.

Table Movement

Craniocaudal.

Reconstruction Kernel/Algorithm

Use a high-resolution reconstruction algorithm.

Window Level (WL)/Window Width (WW)

Approximate setting for:

- Lung window: –600 HU = WL; +1500 HU = WW (Figures 19–2 and 19–3)

SPECIAL CONSIDERATIONS

The mAs may need to be increased due to increased noise on images with thinner slice thickness.

Multiplanar Reconstruction (MPR)

Using an axial image, position the slice overlay to produce coronal MPR images and position vertically to produce sagittal MPR images. For sagittal images, use an odd number of slices and align the middle slice along the midline of the body to produce a midline sagittal image.

Contrast Media

No intravenous (IV) contrast media is needed.

Radiation Reduction Options

- Use automatic tube modulation with the patient's arms raised above their head. If IV contrast is being used, place the IV prior to positioning.
- Use iterative reconstruction technique.

20
CT Angiography (CTA) Chest: Pulmonary Emboli (PE)

INDICATIONS

Pulmonary thromboembolism, commonly called a pulmonary embolism (PE), is an occlusion of the pulmonary arterial system. Pulmonary CT angiography (CTA) is the modality of choice for acute PE.

IMAGING APPLICATIONS

Patient/Part Positioning

Position the patient supine and headfirst in the gantry. Adjust the patient so they are straight and flat (no rotation of the body) on the table. After an intravenous (IV) line is in place, position the patient's arms above their head. If needed, support the patient's arms on a pillow above their head. This is to be performed prior to acquiring the anteroposterior (AP) and lateral scout images (Figure 20–1A).

Breathing Instructions

Inspiration breath hold.

Scan Range

Use AP (Figure 20–1B) and lateral scouts to assist with the placement of the slice overlay for axial images. Extend the slice overlay from the thoracic inlet (located just above the apex of the lung) inferiorly to include the adrenal glands. See Figures 20–2 and 20–3.

Gantry Angulation

Gantry angulation is 0 degrees.

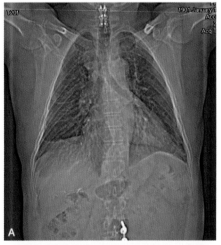
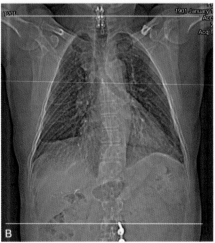

FIGURE 20–1. (A) AP scout of the chest. **(B)** AP scout of the chest with slice overlay showing the scan range and axial slice orientation indicated by the superiorly and inferiorly placed lines.

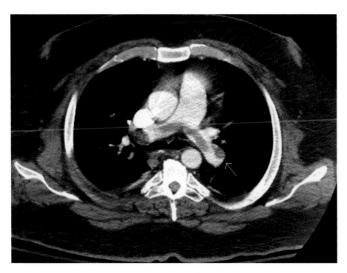

FIGURE 20–2. Axial CT with IV contrast at the level of the pulmonary trunk and left and right pulmonary arteries. The hypodense areas within the pulmonary arteries are the pulmonary emboli causing the filling defect.

Field of View

The field of view should be large enough to include the patient's chest region.

Slice Thickness

Reconstructed slice thickness of 5 to 8 mm is commonly used. A slice thickness of 3 mm or less provides better spatial resolution.

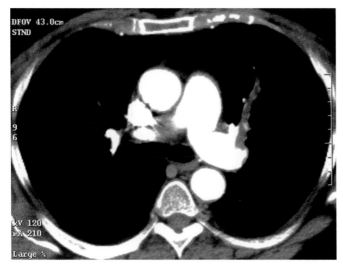

FIGURE 20–3. Axial CT with IV contrast showing filling defect in a branch coming off the left pulmonary artery. (Reprinted from Grey ML, Alinani JM. *CT and MRI Pathology: A Pocket Atlas*. McGraw-Hill; 2018, with permission from The McGraw-Hill Companies.)

Table Movement

Caudocranial direction of scanning ensures adequate contrast material in the lower pulmonary vessels and minimizes streak artifact from contrast in the superior vena cava (SVC) or brachiocephalic vein.

Reconstruction Kernel/Algorithm

Soft tissue and lung algorithms.

Window Level (WL)/Window Width (WW)

Approximate setting for:

- Soft tissue window: +40 HU = WL; +400 HU = WW
- Lung window: –200 HU = WL; +2000 HU = WW
- Bone window: +300 HU = WL; +1500 HU = WW

Contrast Media

IV contrast–enhanced exam with bolus tracking is suggested. Place the region of interest in the pulmonary trunk or main pulmonary artery. Typically, 60 to 150 mL of IV contrast is administered at a rate of 5 mL/s, followed by a saline chaser at the same rate to allow washout of the contrast from the SVC, thus minimizing streak artifact.

Complete occlusions or partial occlusions present as filling defects in the periphery of the affected vessel.

SPECIAL CONSIDERATIONS

- Triple-rule-out CT examination uses an electrocardiogram-synchronized acquisition throughout the entire chest with the aim of excluding 3 major causes of acute chest pain: (1) PE, (2) acute aortic syndrome, and (3) acute coronary syndrome.
- Coronal and sagittal multiplanar reconstruction (MPR), if requested

Radiation Reduction Options

- Use automatic tube modulation.
- Use iterative reconstruction technique.

HISTORICAL NOTE

Ventilation-perfusion scintigraphy (V/Q) scanning used to be the first-line test in stable patients. Current CT technology is faster and produces better-quality images with less radiation exposure than V/Q scanning.

21
Chest Trauma

INDICATIONS

Used to evaluate the following:

- Penetrating trauma to the thorax such as gunshot and stab injuries
- Suspected mediastinal injury, specifically the great vessels; for example, in rapid deceleration usually during a motor vehicle accident
- Pneumothorax, contusion, laceration, abnormal cardio-mediastinal contour, rib fractures, and foreign bodies

IMAGING APPLICATIONS

Patient/Part Positioning

Position the patient supine and headfirst in the gantry. Adjust the patient so they are straight and flat (no rotation of the body) on the table. After an intravenous (IV) line is in place, the patient's arms will be positioned above their head. If needed, support the patient's arms on a pillow above their head; however, depending on the status of the patient, they may need to leave their arms by their side. This is to be performed prior to acquiring the anteroposterior (AP) and lateral scout images (Figure 21–1A).

Breathing Instructions

If possible, suspended inspiration.

Scan Range

Use AP and lateral (Figure 21–1B) scouts to assist with the placement of the slice overlay for axial images. Extend the slice overlay from the thoracic outlet (located just above the apex of the lung) through the lung to the level of the adrenal glands. See Figures 21–2, 21–3, and 21–4.

Gantry Angulation

No gantry angle is needed.

Field of View

The field of view should be large enough to include the patient's chest region.

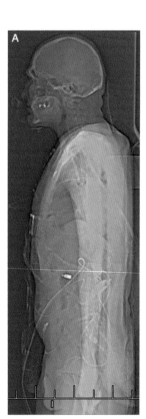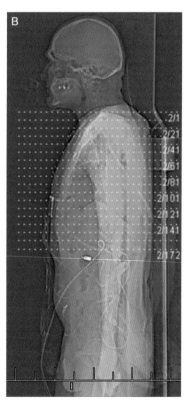

FIGURE 21-1. **(A)** Lateral scout image. Trauma situations may require a longer scout image to then set up multiple exams that are tailored to the specific anatomic region of the body. **(B)** In this case, the chest area shows the slice overlay covering the extent of the chest region.

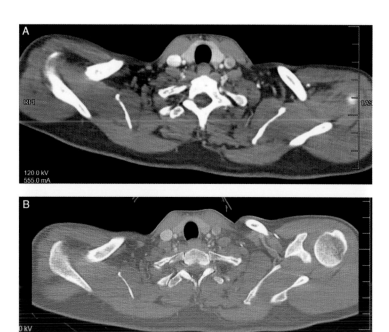

FIGURE 21-2. Axial CT at the upper level of the chest examination. **(A)** Mediastinal window. **(B)** Lung window. Note that the fracture of the first rib on the right side is better seen in Figure 2B.

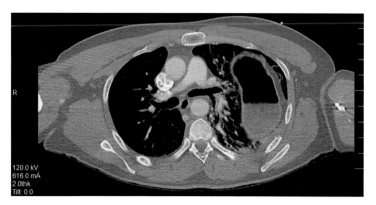

FIGURE 21-3. Axial image showing the herniation of the stomach through the diaphragm into the thoracic cavity. Note the air-fluid level within the stomach.

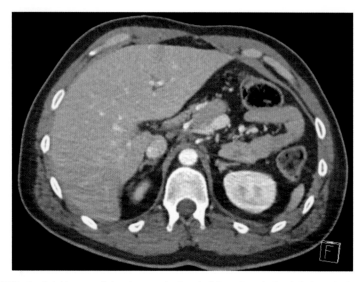

FIGURE 21-4. Axial image of the chest at the level of the adrenal glands below the herniation.

Slice Thickness

Reconstructed slice thickness of 5 to 8 mm is commonly used.

Table Movement

Craniocaudal.

Reconstruction Kernel/Algorithm

Soft tissue and lung algorithms. Bone window may be helpful in trauma cases.

Window Level (WL)/Window Width (WW)

Approximate setting for:

- Soft tissue window: +40 HU = WL; +400 HU = WW
- Lung window: –200 HU = WL; +2000 HU = WW
- Bone window: +300 HU = WL; +1500 HU = WW

SPECIAL CONSIDERATIONS

- Multiplanar reconstruction (MPR)
  - Coronal MPR to the body axis. See Figure 21–5.
  - Sagittal MPR to the body axis. See Figure 21–6.
- Place bolus triggering in the ascending aorta if using IV contrast.

Contrast Media

IV contrast enhanced. See Chapter 18.

Radiation Reduction Options

- Use automatic tube modulation.
- Use iterative reconstruction technique.

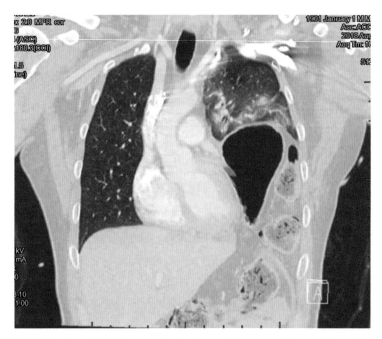

FIGURE 21–5. Coronal MPR showing the herniation of the stomach into the thoracic cavity.

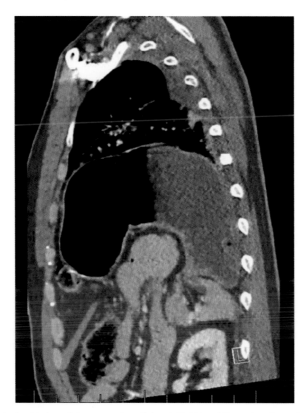

FIGURE 21–6. Parasagittal MPR showing the herniation of the stomach and the air-fluid level. Note that the patient is positioned supine.

22
Routine Abdomen and Pelvis

INDICATIONS

Pain, urinary calculi, appendicitis, suspected mass, primary and metastatic malignancies, complications following surgery, bowel obstruction, guidance for interventional or therapeutic procedures, radiation therapy treatment planning, pre- and posttransplant assessment, and vascular assessment.

IMAGING APPLICATIONS

Patient/Part Positioning

Position the patient supine and headfirst in the gantry. Adjust the patient so they are straight and flat (no rotation of the body) on the table. After an intravenous (IV) line is in place, the patient's arms will be positioned above their head. If needed, support the patient's arms on a pillow above their head. This is to be performed prior to acquiring the anteroposterior (AP) and lateral scout images (Figure 22–1A).

Breathing Instructions

Exhalation. If the patient is unable to hold their breath during the scan, shallow breathing may be helpful.

Scan Range

Use AP and lateral scouts to assist with the placement of the slice overlay for axial images. Extend the slice overlay from a point just above the diaphragm through to the ischial tuberosity. See Figure 22–1B.

Gantry Angulation

Gantry angulation is 0 degrees.

Field of View

The field of view should be large enough to include the patient's body.

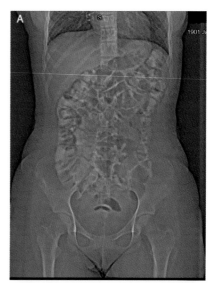
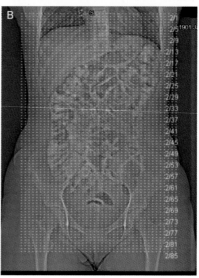

FIGURE 22–1. AP scout of the abdomen and pelvis **(A)** and with slice overlay showing the scan range and axial slice orientation indicated by the superiorly and inferiorly placed lines **(B)**.

Slice Thickness

Reconstructed slice thickness of 5 to 8 mm is commonly used. A slice thickness of 3 mm or less provides better spatial resolution.

Table Movement

Craniocaudal.

Reconstruction Kernel/Algorithm

Soft tissue and lung algorithms. Bone window may be helpful in trauma cases.

Window Level (WL)/Window Width (WW)

Approximate setting for:

- Soft tissue window: +50 HU = WL; +350 HU = WW
- Lung window: −200 HU = WL; +2000 HU = WW
- Bone window: +300 HU = WL; +1500 HU = WW

SPECIAL CONSIDERATIONS

- Multiplanar reconstruction (MPR): Using an axial image, position the slice overlay to produce coronal MPR images and position vertical to produce sagittal MPR images. For the sagittal images, use an odd number of slices and align the middle slice along the midline of the body to have a midline sagittal.

- IV contrast enhancement during various phases of blood circulation can help improve lesion detection and narrow the differential diagnosis (Figures 22–2, A-D, 22–3, and 22–4, A-C).

- CT angiography of the abdomen and pelvis: Place bolus triggering (bolus tracking) ROI in the aorta proximal

- Three-dimensional shaded surface display (SSD) and volume rendered (VR) data reconstruction of the gastrointestinal tract may be helpful in evaluating disease.

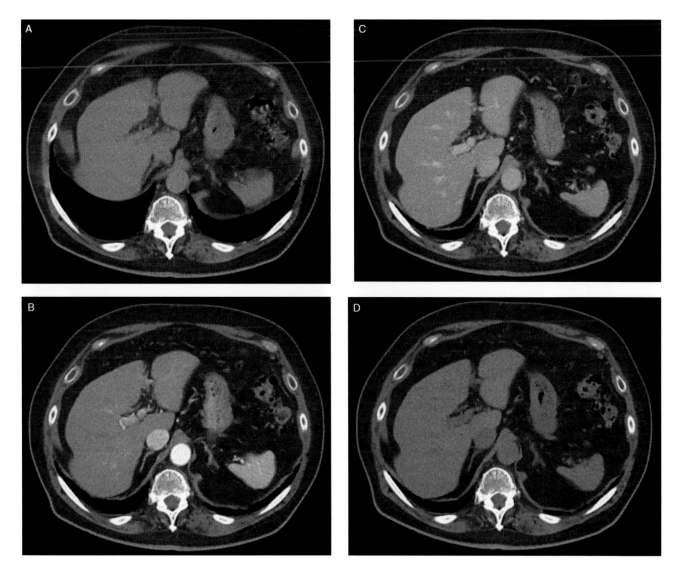

FIGURE 22–2. Axial images at the same level showing noncontrast **(A)**, arterial phase **(B)**, venous phase **(C)**, and 10-minute delay **(D)**.

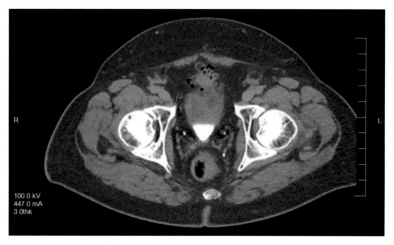

FIGURE 22–3. Axial image at 10-minute delay showing filling of the urinary bladder.

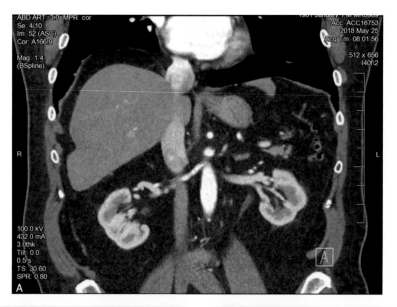

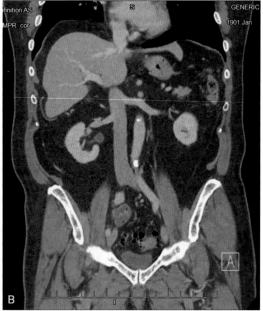

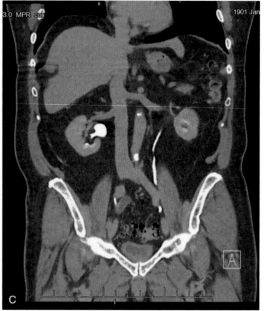

FIGURE 22–4. Coronal MPR images in the arterial phase **(A)**, venous phase **(B)**, and 10-minute delay **(C)**.

Contrast Media

Depending on the physician's order, most exams will require IV contrast and possibly oral contrast media to be used. Dilute barium sulfate, water, or air may be used as the oral contrast agent. If there is suspected perforation of the bowel, Gastrografin may be used. For patients requiring oral contrast, it is suggested that the patient fast at least 6 hours prior to the exam.

No IV contrast is used when evaluating for urolithiasis (kidney stone) or suspected abdominal hemorrhage.

Radiation Reduction Options

- Use automatic tube modulation with patient's arms raised above their head. If IV contrast is being used, place the IV catheter prior to positioning the patient's arms.
- Use iterative reconstruction technique.

23

CTA Vascular Abdomen and Pelvis (AAA)

INDICATIONS

CT angiography (CTA) of the abdomen and pelvis is designed to focus on evaluating the vascular structures in the abdomen and pelvis. Indications include aneurysm, stenosis, ischemia, trauma, and postoperative complications.

IMAGING APPLICATIONS

Patient/Part Positioning

Position the patient supine and headfirst in the gantry. Adjust the patient so they are straight and flat (no rotation of the body) on the table. After an intravenous (IV) line is in place, the patient's arms will be positioned above their head. If needed, support the patient's arms on a pillow above their head. This is to be performed prior to acquiring the anteroposterior (AP) (Figure 23–1A) and lateral scout images.

Scan Range

Use AP (Figure 23–1B) and lateral scouts to assist with the placement of the slice overlay for axial images. Extend the slice overlay from a point just above the diaphragm through to the ischial tuberosity. See Figures 23–2 and 23–3.

Gantry Angulation

Gantry angulation is 0 degrees.

Slice Thickness

Thin-section images (3 mm or less) provide increased spatial resolution.

Table Movement

Craniocaudal.

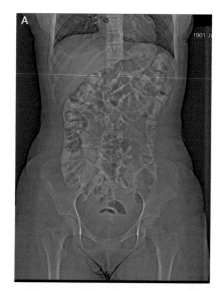

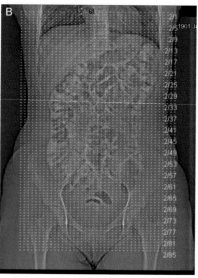

FIGURE 23–1. **(A)** AP scout of the abdomen and pelvis, and **(B)** slice overlay showing the scan range and axial slice orientation indicated by the superiorly and inferiorly placed lines.

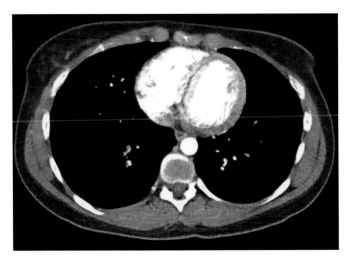

FIGURE 23–2. Axial image with IV contrast at the superior level of the scan range.

Reconstruction Kernel/Algorithm

Soft tissue and lung algorithms. Bone window may be helpful in trauma cases.

Window Level (WL)/Window Width (WW)

Approximate setting for:

- Soft tissue window: +50 HU = WL; +350 HU = WW
- Lung window: –200 HU = WL; +2000 HU = WW
- Bone window: +300 HU = WL; +1500 HU = WW

Contrast Media

IV contrast injection is critical for a CTA procedure. Key considerations include the injected volume of the contrast agent, flow rate, and scan delay. Other important factors are injection site (cubital vein access), large-bore IV catheter (eg, 18 gauge), and saline flush (volume in milliliters). These factors should be adapted to the clinical imaging task.

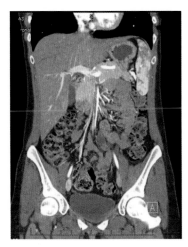

FIGURE 23–4. Coronal MPR image showing branches of the superior mesenteric artery and external iliac arteries.

SPECIAL CONSIDERATIONS

- Place bolus triggering (bolus tracking) region of interest (ROI) in the descending aorta.
- Three-dimensional shaded surface display (SSD) and volume rendered (VR) data reconstruction of the gastrointestinal tract may be helpful in evaluating disease.
- Multiplanar reconstruction (MPR): Using an axial image, position the slice overlay to produce coronal MPR images (Figure 23–4) and position vertically to produce sagittal MPR images. For the sagittal images, use an odd number of slices and align the middle slice along the midline of the body to have a midline sagittal. See Figure 23–5.

Radiation Reduction

- Use automatic tube modulation with the patient's arms raised above their head. Place the IV prior to positioning.
- Use iterative reconstruction technique.

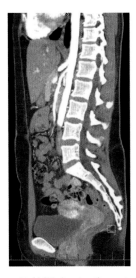

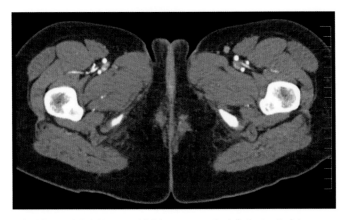

FIGURE 23–3. Axial image with IV contrast at the inferior level of the scan range.

FIGURE 23–5. Midline sagittal MPR showing the aorta. Branching anteriorly off the abdominal aorta are the celiac artery and the superior mesenteric artery.

24

Abdomen and Pelvis Trauma

INDICATIONS

Polytrauma, blunt trauma, suspected fractures, and internal injuries.

IMAGING APPLICATIONS

Patient/Part Positioning

Position the patient supine and headfirst in the gantry. Adjust the patient so they are straight and flat (no rotation of the body) on the table. After an intravenous (IV) line is in place, position the patient's arms above their head. If needed, support the patient's arms on a pillow above their head. This is to be performed prior to acquiring the AP and lateral scout images (Figure 24–1A).

Breathing Instructions

Exhalation. If the patient is unable to hold their breath during the scan, shallow breathing may be helpful.

Scan Range

Use anteroposterior (AP) and lateral (Figure 24–1B) scouts to assist with the placement of the slice overlay for axial images. Extend the slice overlay from a point just above the diaphragm through to the ischial tuberosity (Figure 24–2).

Gantry Angulation

No gantry angle is needed.

Field of View

The field of view should be large enough to include the patient's body.

Slice Thickness

Reconstructed slice thickness of 5 to 8 mm is commonly used.

Table Movement

Craniocaudal.

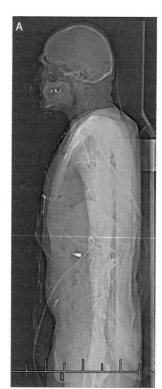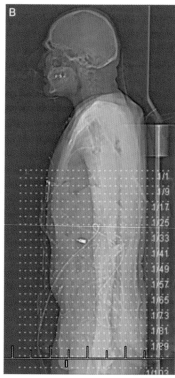

FIGURE 24–1. Lateral scout of the abdomen and pelvis **(A)**, and with slice overlay showing the scan range and axial slice orientation indicated by the superiorly and inferiorly placed lines **(B)**.

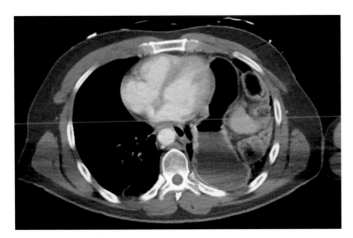

FIGURE 24–2. Axial image showing the stomach herniated through the diaphragm into the thoracic cavity.

Reconstruction Kernel/Algorithm

Soft tissue and lung algorithms. Bone window may be helpful in trauma cases.

Window Level (WL)/Window Width (WW)

Approximate setting for:

- Soft tissue window: +50 HU = WL; +350 HU = WW
- Lung window: –200 HU = WL; +2000 HU = WW
- Bone window: +300 HU = WL; +1500 HU = WW

SPECIAL CONSIDERATIONS

- Multiplanar reconstruction (MPR): Position the slice overlay to produce coronal and sagittal MPRs. See Figure 24–3.
- Shaded surface display may be helpful to evaluate fractures.
- Volume rendering may be helpful in the evaluation of vascular structures.

Contrast Media

IV contrast is helpful in evaluating blunt abdominal or flank trauma. Retrograde filling of the bladder may be useful in evaluating for bladder injury.

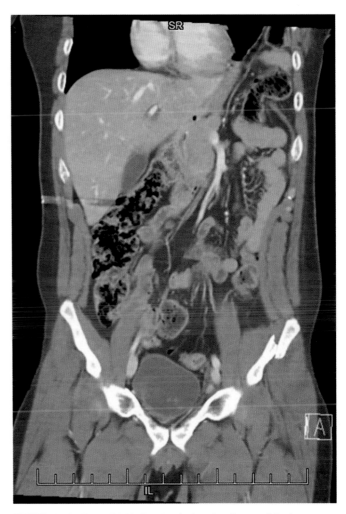

FIGURE 24–3. Coronal MPR showing the herniated stomach in the thoracic cavity.

Radiation Reduction Options

- Use automatic tube modulation with the patient's arms raised above their head (if possible). If IV contrast is being used, the IV catheter should be inserted prior to positioning the patient's arms.
- Use iterative reconstruction technique.

25
Liver (Multi-Phasic)

INDICATIONS

Lesions of the liver such as hepatocellular carcinoma (HCC), focal nodular hyperplasia, adenoma, and hemangioma.

IMAGING APPLICATIONS

Patient/Part Positioning

Position the patient supine and headfirst in the gantry. Adjust the patient so they are straight and flat (no rotation of the body) on the table. After an intravenous (IV) line is in place, the patient's arms will be positioned above their head. If needed, support the patient's arms on a pillow above their head. This is to be performed prior to acquiring the anteroposterior (AP) (Figure 25–1A) and lateral scout images.

Breathing Instructions

Full Inspiration.

Scan Range

Use AP and lateral scouts to assist with the placement of the slice overlay for axial images. Extend the slice overlay from the diaphragm inferiorly to the iliac crest. See Figure 25–1B.

Gantry Angulation

Gantry angulation is 0 degrees.

Slice Thickness

Use a slice thickness of 5 mm or less. Thinner slice thickness improves spatial resolution and improves detail of multiplanar reconstructions (MPRs).

Table Movement

Craniocaudal.

Reconstruction Kernel/Algorithm

Soft tissue algorithm.

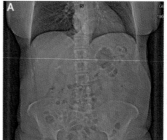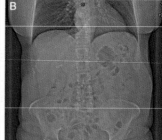

FIGURE 25–1. AP scout of the abdomen and pelvis **(A)**, and with slice overlay showing the scan range and axial slice orientation indicated by the superiorly and inferiorly placed lines **(B)**.

WL/WW

Approximate setting for:

- Soft tissue window: +50 HU = WL; +350 HU = WW

Contrast Media

IV contrast for triple-phase protocol includes: (1) late arterial phase (15-30 seconds after bolus trigger or 35-45 seconds following the injection); (2) portal venous phase (60-75 seconds after injection), and (3) delayed phase (2-5 minutes following injection). Note: A 4-phase liver protocol would include a non-enhanced liver (Figure 25–2) and then the triple phase.

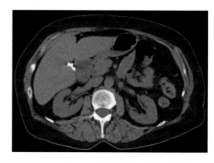

FIGURE 25–2. Axial nonenhanced CT of liver after cholecystectomy. Figures 25–2 to 25–4 are at the same level.

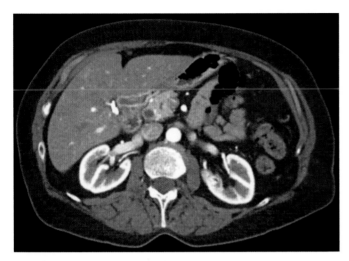

FIGURE 25–3. Axial CT image of liver in the arterial phase postcholecystectomy.

Place bolus tracking region of interest (ROI) in the aorta at the level of the diaphragmatic hiatus or L1 vertebra. Set the threshold at 150 HU.

1. Late arterial phase (Figure 25–3)
   - Portal vein is enhanced.
   - There is no hepatic vein enhancement.
   - HCC may only show enhancement.
2. Portal venous phase (Figure 25–4)
   - Portal veins are enhanced.
   - Hepatic veins are enhanced.
3. Delayed phase
   - Portal and hepatic veins are slightly enhanced.

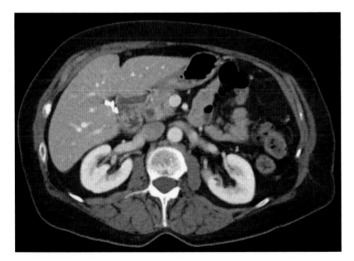

FIGURE 25–4. Axial CT image of liver in the venous phase postcholecystectomy.

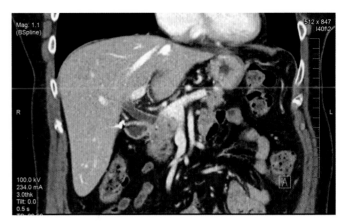

FIGURE 25–5. Coronal MPR in the venous phase.

SPECIAL CONSIDERATIONS

- MPR: Using an axial image, position the slice overlay to produce coronal MPR images (Figure 25–5) and position vertical to produce sagittal MPR images (Figure 25–6). For the sagittal images, use an odd number of slices and align the middle slice along the midline of the body to have a midline sagittal.

Radiation Reduction

- Use automatic tube modulation with the patient's arms raised above their head. If IV contrast is being used, the IV catheter should be inserted prior to positioning.
- Use iterative reconstruction technique.

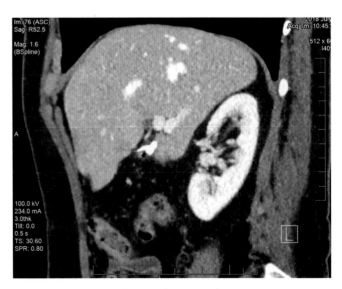

FIGURE 25–6. Parasagittal MPR in the venous phase.

26

Adrenal Glands

INDICATIONS

To further evaluate incidentally discovered adrenal lesions and to identify adrenal abnormalities when clinically suspected.

IMAGING APPLICATIONS

Patient/Part Positioning

Position the patient supine and headfirst in the gantry. Adjust the patient so they are straight and flat (no rotation of the body) on the table. After an intravenous (IV) line is in place, the patient's arms will be positioned above their head. If needed, support the patient's arms on a pillow above their head. This is to be performed prior to acquiring the anteroposterior (AP) (Figure 26–1A) and lateral scout images.

Breathing Instructions

Inspiration.

Scan Range

Use AP (Figure 26–1B) and lateral scouts to assist with the placement of the slice overlay for axial images. Extend the slice overlay from a point just above the diaphragm to the iliac crest.

Gantry Angulation

Gantry angulation is 0 degrees.

Slice Thickness

For malignant diseases, a slice thickness of 5 mm may be used. For detecting small endocrine tumors, a thin-slice thickness of 3 mm or less is helpful.

Table Movement

Craniocaudal.

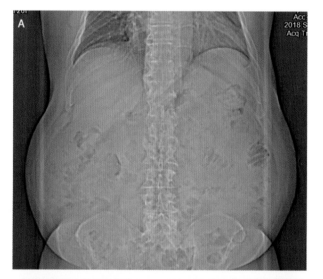

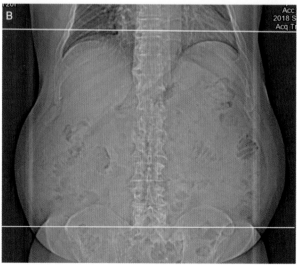

FIGURES 26–1. AP scout of the abdomen **(A)**, with slice overlay showing the scan range and axial slice orientation indicated by the superiorly and inferiorly placed lines **(B)**.

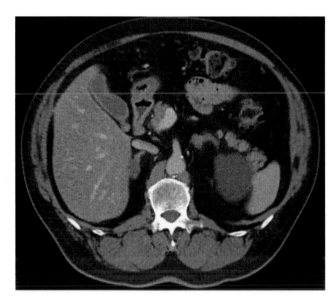

FIGURES 26–2. Axial image with IV contrast several slices down from the superior level. This image is at the level of the celiac artery.

Reconstruction Kernel/Algorithm

Soft tissue algorithm.

Window Level (WL)/Window Width (WW)

Approximate setting for:

- Noncontrast window: +40 HU = WL; +300 HU = WW
- Contrast enhanced: +70 HU = WL; +400 HU = WW

Contrast Media

IV contrast is used to help differentiate between adenomas and nonadenomas. Baseline exam is noncontrast followed by an IV contrast-enhanced scan in portal venous phase (60-70 seconds after injection) (Figures 26–2 to 26–4) followed by a delayed scan at 15 minutes.

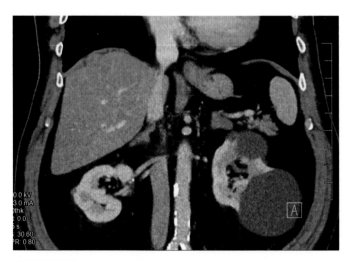

FIGURES 26–3. Coronal MPR showing multiple cystic lesions on the left kidney and another very small cystic lesion on the right kidney. Hard plaque is seen in the abdominal aorta. Cross-sections of the celiac and superior mesenteric arteries are also seen. The adrenal gland is seen on the right side.

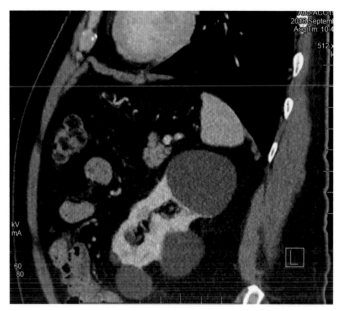

FIGURES 26–4. Sagittal MPR showing cystic lesions on the left kidney.

Arterial phase is helpful in distinguishing adrenals from adjacent structures. Arterial phase may not contribute to the differential diagnosis of benign versus malignant lesions. Delayed scanning 15 minutes post IV injection is helpful in differentiating adenomas from nonadenomas.

SPECIAL CONSIDERATIONS

Multiplanar Reconstruction (MPR)

Using an axial image, position the slice overlay to produce coronal MPR images (Figure 26–3) and position vertical to produce sagittal MPR images (Figure 26–4). For the sagittal images, use an odd number of slices and align the middle slice along the midline of the body to have a midline sagittal.

Radiation Reduction

- Use automatic tube modulation with the patient's arms raised above their head. If IV contrast is being used, the IV catheter should be inserted prior to positioning the patient's arms.
- Use iterative reconstruction technique.

27

CT Urography: Urolithiasis (Stone)

INDICATIONS

To evaluate for renal/ureter calculi.

IMAGING APPLICATIONS

Patient/Part Positioning

Position the patient supine and head first in the gantry. Adjust the patient so they are straight and flat (no rotation of the body) on the table. Position the patient's arms above their head. If needed, support the patient's arms on a pillow above their head. This is to be performed prior to acquiring the anteroposterior (AP) (Figure 27–1A) and lateral scout images.

Breathing Instructions

Suspended inspiration.

Scan Range

Use AP and lateral scouts to assist with the placement of the slice overlay for axial images. Extend the slice overlay from a point just above the diaphragm through to the ischial tuberosity. See Figure 27–1B.

Gantry Angulation

Gantry angulation is 0 degrees.

Field of View

The field of view should be large enough to include the patient's abdomen and pelvis.

Slice Thickness

Reconstructed slice thickness of 5 to 8 mm is commonly used.

Table Movement

Craniocaudal.

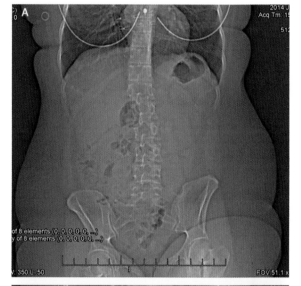

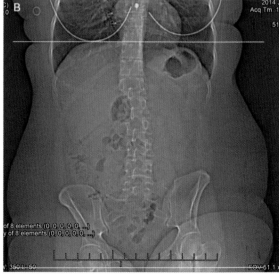

FIGURE 27–1. AP scout of the abdomen and pelvis **(A)**, and with slice overlay showing the scan range and axial slice orientation indicated by the superiorly and inferiorly placed lines **(B)**.

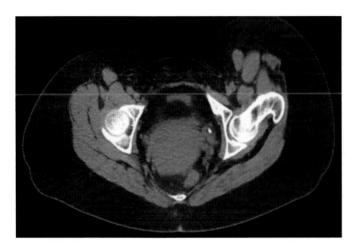

FIGURE 27-2. Axial noncontrast image showing a stone in the left ureter in the pelvic area.

Reconstruction Kernel/Algorithm

Soft tissue algorithm should be used.

Window Level (WL)/Window Width (WW)

Approximate setting for:

- Soft tissue window: +50 HU = WL; +350 HU = WW

SPECIAL CONSIDERATIONS

Contrast Media

No IV contrast media is needed. See Figure 27–2.

Multiplanar Reconstruction (MPR)

Using an axial image, position the slice overlay to produce coronal MPR images (Figure 27–3) and position vertical to produce sagittal MPR images. For the sagittal images, use an odd

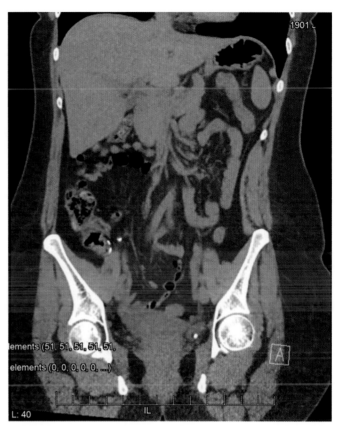

FIGURE 27-3. Coronal MPR showing the stone in the left ureter of the pelvis.

number of slices and align the middle slice along the midline of the body to have a midline sagittal.

Radiation Reduction Options

- Use automatic tube modulation.
- Use iterative reconstruction technique.

28

Renal CT Angiography (CTA)

INDICATIONS

Renal artery stenosis, atherosclerotic disease, and fibromuscular dysplasia of the renal arteries.

IMAGING APPLICATIONS

Patient/Part Positioning

Position the patient supine and headfirst in the gantry. Adjust the patient so they are straight and flat (no rotation of the body) on the table. After an intravenous (IV) line is in place, the patient's arms will be positioned above their head. If needed, support the patient's arms on a pillow above their head. This is to be performed prior to acquiring the anteroposterior (AP) (Figure 28–1A) and lateral scout images.

Breathing Instructions

Full Inspiration.

Scan Range

Use AP and lateral scouts to assist with the placement of the slice overlay for axial images. Extend the slice overlay from a point just above the diaphragm through to the ischial crest. See Figure 28–1B.

Gantry Angulation

Gantry angulation is 0 degrees.

Field of View

The field of view should be large enough to include the patient's body.

Slice Thickness

Thin-section (≤5 mm) axial images. Thin axial images will improve the quality of coronal multiplanar reconstruction (MPR) and curved planar reformats.

Table Movement

Craniocaudal.

Reconstruction Kernel/Algorithm

Soft tissue algorithm.

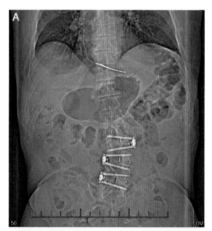
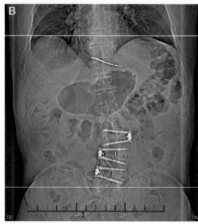

FIGURE 28–1. AP scout of the abdomen **(A)**, with slice overlay showing the scan range and axial slice orientation indicated by the superiorly and inferiorly placed lines **(B)**.

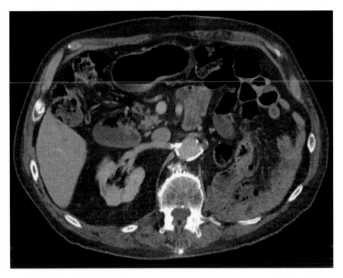

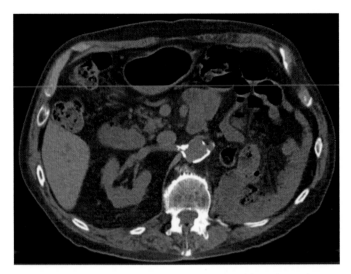

FIGURE 28-2. Noncontrast axial image at the level of the right renal artery. Figures 28-2 to 28-4 are at the same level. Note that this patient has had a nephrectomy of their left kidney.

FIGURE 28-4. Venous phase.

- Nephrogenic or venous phase: 55- to 65-second delay (Figure 28-4)
- Excretory phase: 5-minute delay

Window Level (WL)/Window Width (WW)

Approximate setting for:

- Soft tissue window: +50 HU = WL; +350 HU = WW

SPECIAL CONSIDERATIONS

- MPR: Using an axial image, position the slice overlay to produce thin coronal MPR (Figure 28-5).
- Curved MPR of the renal artery.

Contrast Media

IV contrast is used with a 4- to 5-mL/s injection rate to better visualize the vascular structures. For bolus tracking, place the region of interest (ROI) in the aorta at the level of the diaphragm. A 4-phase CT angiography (CTA) of the kidney would include:

- Noncontrast phase (Figure 28-2)
- Arterial or corticomedullary phase: 25- to 30-second delay (Figure 28-3)

Radiation Reduction

- Use automatic tube modulation with the patient's arms raised above their head. If IV contrast is being used, the IV catheter should be inserted prior to positioning the patient's arms.
- Use iterative reconstruction technique.

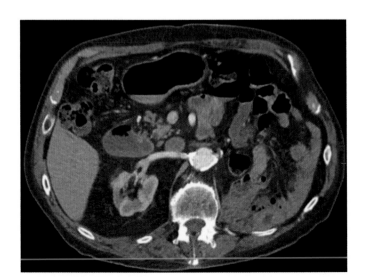

FIGURE 28-3. Arterial phase.

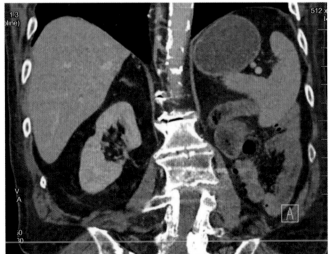

FIGURE 28-5. Coronal MPR.

29

Pancreas

INDICATIONS

Jaundice, pancreatic diseases, tumor and cystic lesion assessment, pancreatitis, and CT-guided biopsy or drainage.

IMAGING APPLICATIONS

Patient/Part Positioning

Position the patient supine and headfirst in the gantry. Adjust the patient so they are straight and flat (no rotation of the body) on the table. After an intravenous (IV) line is in place, the patient's arms will be positioned above their head. If needed, support the patient's arms on a pillow above their head. This is to be performed prior to acquiring the anteroposterior (AP) (Figure 29–1A) and lateral scout images.

Breathing Instructions

Inspiration.

Scan Range

Use AP and lateral scouts to assist with the placement of the slice overlay for axial images. Extend the slice overlay from a point just above the diaphragm through to the iliac crest or symphysis pubis. See Figure 29–1B.

- Arterial phase: Diaphragm to iliac crest
- Venous phase: Diaphragm to iliac crest, maybe entire pelvis

Gantry Angulation

Gantry angulation is 0 degrees.

Slice Thickness

Use thin slice thickness for better spatial resolution and for multiplanar reconstructions (MPRs).

Table Movement

Craniocaudal.

Reconstruction Kernel/Algorithm

Soft tissue and bone windows.

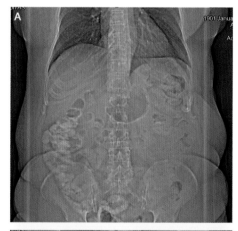

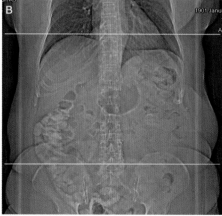

FIGURE 29–1. AP scout of the abdomen and pelvis (**A**), with slice overlay showing the scan range and axial slice orientation indicated by the superiorly and inferiorly placed lines (**B**).

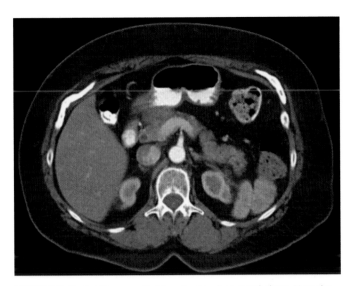

FIGURE 29–2. Axial image with IV contrast in the arterial phase. Note the small hypodense lesion in the head of the pancreas.

Window Level (WL)/Window Width (WW)

Approximate setting for:

- Soft tissue window: +50 HU = WL; +350 HU = WW

Contrast Media

Depending on the physician's order, most exams will require IV contrast and possibly oral contrast (water) to be used. Water (500-1000 mL) may be administered 20 to 30 minutes prior to the exam. IV contrast agent is used to acquire biphasic arterial (Figure 29–2) and venous (Figure 29–3) acquisitions.

Bolus tracking may be used with placement in the abdominal aorta prior to the celiac trunk.

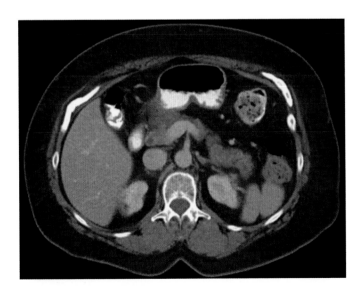

FIGURE 29–3. Same level as above in the venous phase.

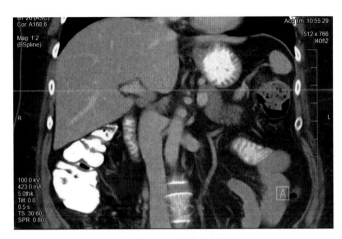

FIGURE 29–4. Coronal MPR showing the body of the pancreas.

SPECIAL CONSIDERATIONS

- MPR: Using an axial image, position the slice overlay to produce coronal MPR images (Figure 29–4) and position vertical to produce sagittal MPR images (Figure 29–5). For the sagittal images, use an odd number of slices and align the middle slice along the midline of the body to have a midline sagittal.
- Dual-energy CT with monochromatic reconstructions.

Radiation Reduction

- Use automatic tube modulation with the patient's arms raised above their head. If IV contrast is being used, the IV catheter should be inserted prior to positioning the patient's arms.
- Use iterative reconstruction technique.

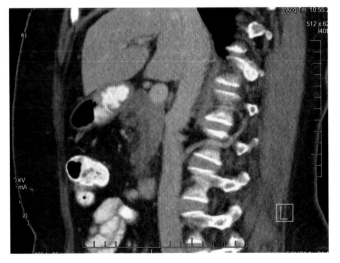

FIGURE 29–5. Parasagittal MPR.

30
Enterography

INDICATIONS

Crohn's disease, small bowel bleeding, suspected small bowel tumor, celiac disease, small bowel obstruction, abdominal pain, and suspected mesenteric ischemia.

IMAGING APPLICATIONS

Patient/Part Positioning

Position the patient supine and headfirst in the gantry. Adjust the patient so they are straight and flat (no rotation of the body) on the table. After an intravenous (IV) line is in place, the patient's arms will be positioned above their head. If needed, support the patient's arms on a pillow above their head. This is to be performed prior to acquiring the anteroposterior (AP) (Figure 30–1A) and lateral scout images.

Breathing Instructions

Full inspiration.

Scan Range

Use AP (Figure 30–1B) and lateral scouts to assist with the placement of the slice overlay for axial images. Extend the slice overlay from a point just above the diaphragm (Figure 30–2) through to the symphysis pubis (Figure 30–3).

Gantry Angulation

Gantry angulation is 0 degrees.

Field of View

The field of view should be large enough to include the patient's body.

Slice Thickness

Thin-section imaging provides better spatial resolution. For multiplanar reconstructions (MPRs), a section thickness of 3 mm or less is recommended.

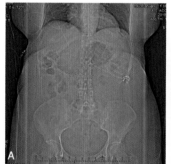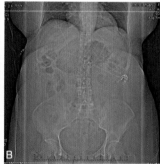

FIGURE 30–1. AP scout of the abdomen and pelvis **(A)**, and with slice overlay showing the scan range and axial slice orientation indicated by the superiorly and inferiorly placed lines **(B)**.

Table Movement

Craniocaudal.

Reconstruction Kernel/Algorithm

Soft tissue window.

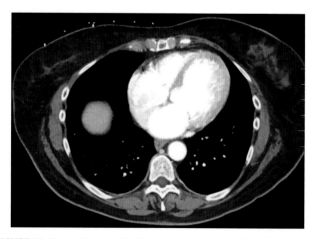

FIGURE 30–2. Axial image with IV contrast at the level of the diaphragm (superior slice).

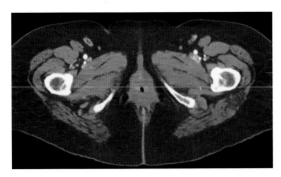

FIGURE 30–3. Axial image at the level of the ischial tuberosity (inferior slice).

Window Level (WL)/Window Width (WW)

Approximate setting for:

- Soft tissue window: +50 HU = WL; +350 HU = WW

Contrast Media

Patient is to be NPO (nothing by mouth) 4 hours before the exam. Oral (negative) contrast with IV contrast and saline bolus at a 4-mL/s injection rate may be used. Arterial and venous phases may be acquired.

SPECIAL CONSIDERATIONS

MPR

Using an axial image, position the slice overlay to produce coronal MPR images (Figure 30–4, A and B) and sagittal MPR images (Figure 30–5).

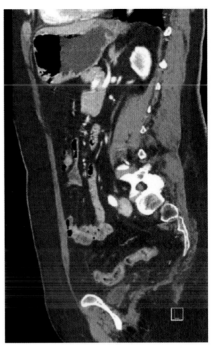

FIGURE 30–5. Parasagittal MPR. Note the air-fluid level in the stomach of this supine patient.

Radiation Reduction

- Use automatic tube modulation with the patient's arms raised above their head. If IV contrast is being used, the IV catheter should be placed prior to positioning the patient's arms.
- Use iterative reconstruction technique.

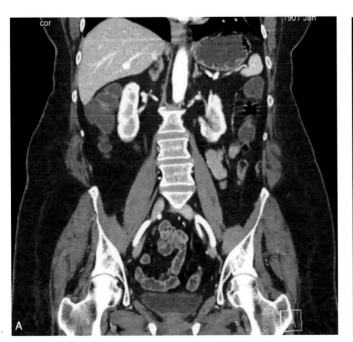

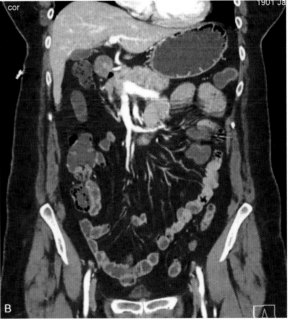

FIGURE 30–4. Coronal MPR images in arterial phase. **A** is slightly posterior to **B**. Note the surrounding anatomic structures such as the psoas muscles, left internal and external iliac arteries **(A)**, and the superior mesenteric artery and its distribution of vessels, and the femoral arteries (bright) and femoral veins just medial to the femoral arteries **(B)**.

31
CT-Guided Biopsy

INDICATIONS

CT may be more useful than other guidance modalities when difficult routes of approach are used. CT-guided biopsy is useful for small focal lesions and for bony or aerated structures.

IMAGING APPLICATIONS

Patient/Part Positioning

Depending on the area/anatomic structure that needs to be biopsied, consult the interventional radiologist performing the procedure on the specific positioning instructions. (See Figure 31–1.)

Breathing Instructions

The interventional radiologist will provide the specific breathing instructions depending on the location of the biopsy.

Scan Range

Consult the interventional radiologist performing the procedure.

Gantry Angulation

Gantry angulation is 0 degrees.

Field of View

The field of view should be large enough to include the patient's body.

Slice Thickness

Use a 5- to 8-mm reconstructed image thickness.

Table Movement

Use axial (step-and-shoot) mode.

Reconstruction Kernel/Algorithm

Soft tissue algorithm should be used. Lung windows will also be used for biopsies in the thoracic cavity.

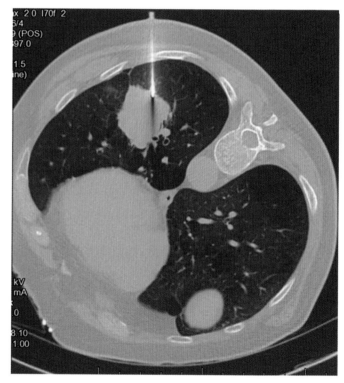

FIGURE 31–1. Following the review of a previous CT exam of the chest, the interventional radiologist selected to scout the patient in a left anterior oblique (LAO) position. The level for the needle biopsy procedure is selected, and the needle is shown in the lesion.

Window Level (WL)/Window Width (WW)

Approximate setting for:

- Soft tissue window: +50 HU = WL; +350 HU = WW
- Lung window: –200 HU = WL; +2000 HU = WW; see Figures 31–1 and 31–2
- Bone window: +300 HU = WL; +1500 HU = WW; see Figure 31–4

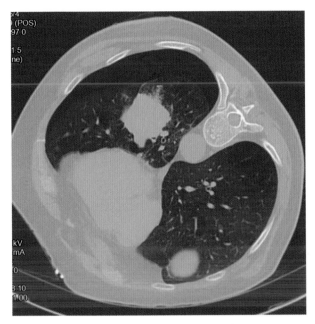

FIGURE 31-2. A pneumothorax is seen following the lung biopsy.

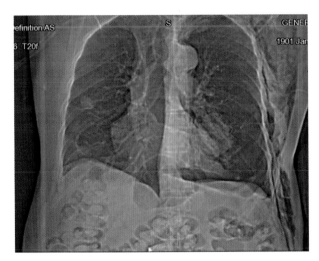

FIGURE 31-3. Anteroposterior scout taken following the lung biopsy in patient shown in Figure 31–2.

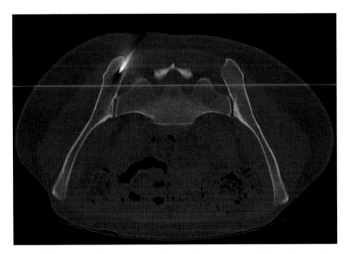

FIGURE 31-4. A different patient than in Figure 31–2 positioned prone for a bone biopsy.

Contrast Media

This is a noncontrast procedure. However, a recent contrast-enhanced study should be available.

SPECIAL CONSIDERATIONS

- Verify labs to monitor clotting factors prior to beginning procedure.
- Monitor for pneumothorax and hemoptysis if biopsy performed on lung. See Figures 31–2 and 31–3.
- Monitor for bleeding.
- Images are saved to document the biopsy procedure.

Radiation Reduction Options

Dose-reduction techniques should be used whenever possible.

- Automatic exposure control
- Iterative reconstruction technique

32
Shoulder

INDICATIONS

Trauma, pain, soft tissue injury, follow-up from a previous injury, bone tumor, presurgery planning, and if an MRI is contraindicated.

IMAGING APPLICATIONS

Patient/Part Positioning

Position the patient supine and headfirst in the gantry. Position the shoulder (if possible) with the arm along the body and the shoulder in a neutral (thumb up) position. The contralateral arm is raised above the head. Stabilize the shoulder to reduce motion artifact.

In addition, positioning the shoulder in an abduction and external rotation (ABER) position may improve detecting partial tears of the rotator cuff when performing CT arthrography.

Scan Range

For axial images, align the slice overlay to be perpendicular to the long axis of the humerus. The scan range extends from the upper acromion (to include the acromioclavicular joint) to the proximal humerus, just below the glenoid (Figures 32–1 and 32–2). If needed, the scan may extend inferiorly to include the distal tip of the scapula.

Gantry Angulation

Gantry angulation is 0 degrees.

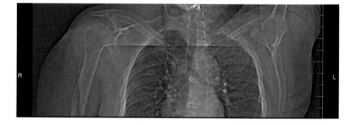

FIGURE 32–1. Anteroposterior scout for right shoulder exam. Note that the left arm is raised above the patient's head to help reduce beam-hardening scatter radiation artifact.

Field of View

Depending on the shoulder anatomy, 22 to 25 cm should cover the anatomic area of interest.

Slice Thickness

Use a reconstructed slice thickness of 3 mm or less for better spatial resolution.

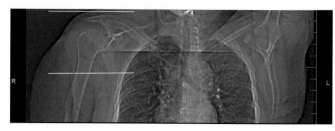

FIGURE 32–2. Anteroposterior scout for right shoulder exam with axial slice overlay.

Table Movement

Craniocaudal.

Reconstruction Algorithm, Filter, or Kernel

Soft tissue and bone algorithms.

Window Level (WL)/Window Width (WW)

Approximate window setting for:

- Soft tissue: +50 HU = WL; +350 HU = WW
- Bone window: +300 HU = WL; +1500 HU = WW

SPECIAL CONSIDERATIONS

- Multiplanar reconstruction (MPR): For a sagittal oblique image, select an axial image that shows the glenoid joint and align the slice overlay to be parallel with the glenoid joint space (Figures 32–3 and 32–4). For a coronal oblique image, select an axial image that shows the glenoid joint and align the slice overlay to be perpendicular to the glenoid joint space (Figures 32–3 and 32–5).
  - Note: Some references may suggest aligning the slice overlay to be parallel to the supraspinous tendon for a coronal oblique image. This may be misleading due to injury. The purpose of imaging the shoulder is to evaluate the joint, so using the glenoid joint to correctly align the slice overlay is recommended.
- Pregnant uterus: According to the American College of Radiology (ACR), if the x-ray beam is properly collimated and the patient is positioned to avoid direct irradiation of

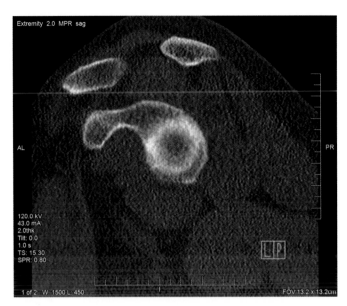

FIGURE 32–4. Sagittal oblique MPR image of the right shoulder.

the pelvis, the amount of exposure to the pregnant uterus would be so low that pregnancy status need not alter the decision to proceed with the examination. However, it is recommended to notify the reading radiologist of a pregnant patient and to obtain the approval to proceed with the examination.

Contrast Media

If ordered as a CT arthrography examination, the direct technique is used to introduce the iodinated contrast media into the joint space under fluoroscopic guidance prior to the CT shoulder examination.

Radiation Reduction Options

- Consider using a thyroid shield.
- Use iterative reconstruction technique.

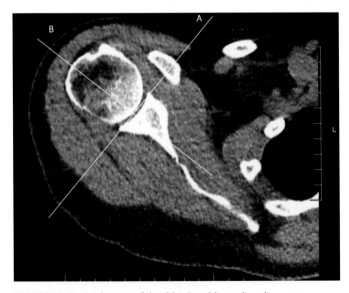

FIGURE 32–3. Axial image of shoulder. For oblique slice alignment, use an axial image showing the glenoid and the head of the shoulder. For the sagittal oblique MPR, align the slice overlay to be (**A**) parallel with the joint. For the coronal oblique MPR, align the slice overlay to be (**B**) perpendicular to the glenoid fossa. For both reconstructions, extend the slice overlay to include the shoulder joint anatomy.

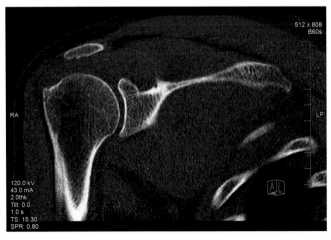

FIGURE 32–5. Coronal oblique MPR image of the right shoulder.

33
Elbow

INDICATIONS

Trauma, fracture or dislocation, pain, soft tissue injury, follow-up from a previous injury, bone tumor, presurgery planning, and if an MRI is contraindicated.

IMAGING APPLICATIONS

Patient/Part Positioning

Position the patient supine and headfirst in the gantry. The elbow may be positioned either by the patient's side or raised above the head with the palm side up. If possible, try to align the elbow straight and along the long axis and in the center of the CT table. However, due to pain or a fracture, positioning the elbow may be challenging and creative. See Figure 33–1.

Stabilize the elbow to reduce motion artifact.

Scan Range

For axial images (Figure 33–2), align the slice overlay to be perpendicular to the long axis of the humerus. The scan range extends from the mid to distal (one-third) humerus just above the epicondyles through to the proximal (one-third) radius/ulna to include the radial tuberosity.

Gantry Angulation

Gantry angulation is 0 degrees.

Field of View

The field of view should be approximately 12 to 15 cm or less. The entire elbow and all related anatomy should be included.

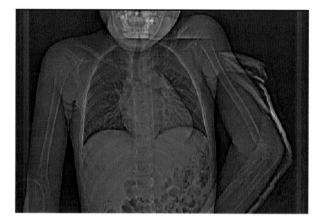

FIGURE 33–1. Anteroposterior scout of patient for left elbow injury. Note that, due to the injury, the patient was unable to straighten their arm.

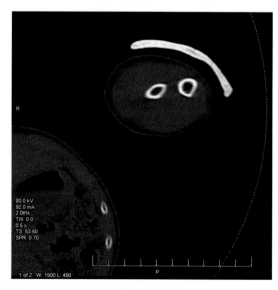

FIGURE 33–2. Axial CT image of forearm.

Slice Thickness

Use a reconstructed slice thickness of 3 mm or less for better spatial resolution.

Table Movement

Caudocranial.

Reconstruction Kernel/Algorithm

Soft tissue and bone algorithms.

Window Level (WL)/Window Width (WW)

Approximate setting for:

- Soft tissue: +50 HU = WL; +350 HU = WW
- Bone window: +300 HU = WL; +1500 HU = WW

SPECIAL CONSIDERATIONS

- Multiplanar reconstruction (MPR): To produce a coronal image, select an axial image and align the slice overlay to be parallel with the epicondyles of the humerus. See Figure 33–3. To produce a sagittal image, select an axial image and align the slice overlay to be perpendicular to the epicondylar plane of the humerus. See Figure 33–4.
- Shaded surface display (SSD) is helpful for fracture and dislocation. See Figure 33–5.
- Intravenous (IV) contrast may be used for tumor or arteriography.

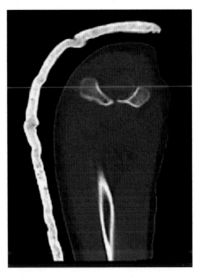

FIGURE 33–4. Sagittal MPR showing fracture of distal humerus.

- CT arthrography examination: The direct technique is used to introduce the iodinated contrast media into the joint space under fluoroscopic guidance prior to the CT shoulder examination.

Contrast Media

There is no IV contrast for a fracture.

Radiation Reduction Options

Positioning the elbow above the head requires a lower radiation dose and increases image quality; however, it might expose the cranium to excessive radiation.

Use the iterative reconstruction technique instead of filtered back-projection to reduce radiation exposure.

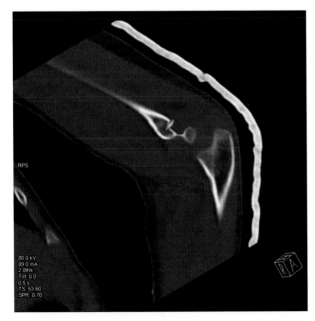

FIGURE 33–3. Coronal MPR.

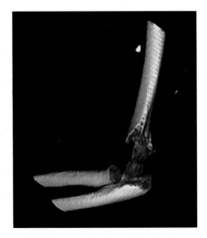

FIGURE 33–5. Three-dimensional shaded surface display (SSD) showing fracture.

34

Wrist

INDICATIONS

Trauma, carpal instability, foreign bodies, pain, soft tissue injury, follow-up from a previous injury, bone tumor, presurgery planning, and if an MRI is contraindicated.

IMAGING APPLICATIONS

Patient/Part Positioning

Position the patient prone and headfirst in the gantry. Position the arm stretched out as straight as possible with the wrist centered in the gantry palm side down. Rest the patient's head on the other arm. See Figures 34–1 and 34–2.

Scan Range

For axial images, scan from the distal metacarpals through to the distal third of the forearm (Figure 34–3).

Gantry Angulation

Gantry angulation is 0 degrees.

Field of View

The field of view should be approximately 15 cm or less. All wrist anatomy should be included.

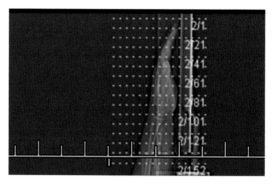

FIGURE 34–2. Lateral scout with slice overlay aligned for axial images.

Slice Thickness

Use a reconstructed slice thickness of 3 mm or less for better spatial resolution.

Table Movement

Craniocaudal.

Reconstruction Kernel/Algorithm

Soft tissue and bone algorithms.

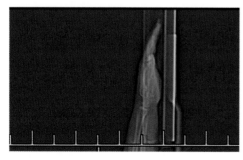

FIGURE 34–1. Lateral scout of the wrist.

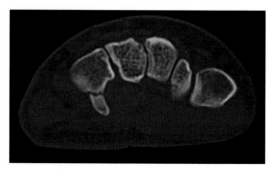

FIGURE 34–3. Axial image of the wrist showing a fracture of the hook of the hamate.

Window Level (WL)/Window Width (WW)

Approximate setting for:

- Soft tissue: +50 HU = WL; +350 HU = WW
- Bone window: +300 HU = WL; +1500 HU = WW

SPECIAL CONSIDERATIONS

Multiplanar Reconstruction

For a coronal image, select an axial image and align the slice overlay to be parallel to the hook of the hamate and the hook of the trapezium (Figure 34–4). For a sagittal image, select an axial image and align the slice overlay to be perpendicular to the hook of the hamate and the hook of the trapezium (Figure 34–5, A and B).

Contrast Media

No contrast is used for bony evaluations.

Radiation Reduction Options

No recommendations.

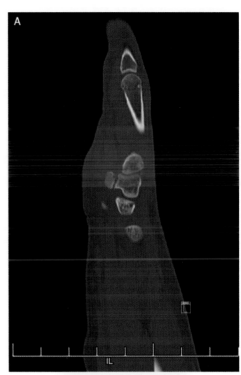
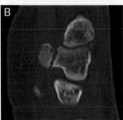

FIGURE 34–5. Sagittal multiplanar reconstruction (MPR) of the wrist (**A**). Note the fracture of the hook of the hamate (**B**) in a magnified image of figure in A.

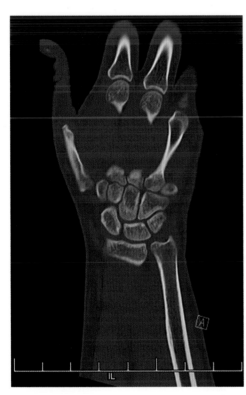

FIGURE 34–4. Coronal multiplanar reconstruction of the wrist.

35
Pelvic Girdle

INDICATIONS

Mostly performed due to trauma.

IMAGING APPLICATIONS

Patient/Part Positioning

Position the patient supine and headfirst in the gantry with their arms above their head. Adjust the patient so they are straight on the table and there is no body rotation. Position the legs flat. If possible, position the pelvis into a true anteroposterior (AP) position with the feet rotated 15 to 20 degrees medially and secured together.

Scan Range

For axial images, align the slice overlay on an AP scout to be parallel to the top of the iliac crest (Figures 35–1 and 35–2). Scan from just above the iliac crest through the ischial tuberosity (Figure 35–2).

Gantry Angulation

Gantry angulation is 0 degrees, parallel with the iliac crest.

Field of View(FOV)

Adjust the FOV to include the entire pelvic area. This may be approximately 40 to 60 cm for teens and adults. For younger children, the FOV may be smaller.

Slice Thickness

Use a reconstructed slice thickness of 3 mm or less for better spatial resolution.

Table Movement

Craniocaudal.

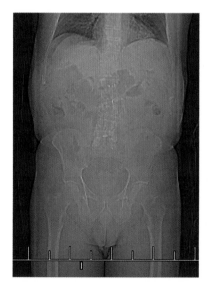

FIGURE 35–1. AP scout for pelvic girdle exam. Note that the patient's arms are positioned above their head.

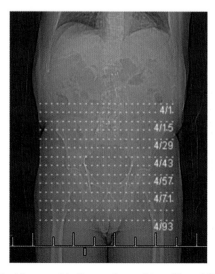

FIGURE 35–2. AP scout with slice overlay positioned for axial images.

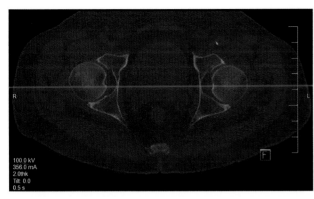

FIGURE 35–3. Axial image. Note the depression on the head of the femur (bilaterally). This is called the fovea capitis. The fovea capitis serves as an attachment point for the ligament of the head of the femur. The older name was ligamentum of teres.

Reconstruction Kernel/Algorithm

Soft tissue and bone algorithms.

Window Level (WL)/Window Width (WW)

Approximate window settings:

- Soft tissue: +50 HU = WL; +350 HU = WW
- Bone window: +300 HU = WL; +1500 HU = WW (see Figure 35–3).

SPECIAL CONSIDERATIONS

- Multiplanar reconstruction (MPR): For coronal images, align the slice overlay to be parallel to the femoral heads. Extend the slice overlay from the ischium through the pubic symphysis (Figure 35–4). For sagittal images,

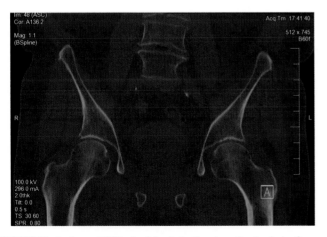

FIGURE 35–4. Coronal MPR of pelvic girdle. Good positioning helps for comparison of left- and right-sided structures.

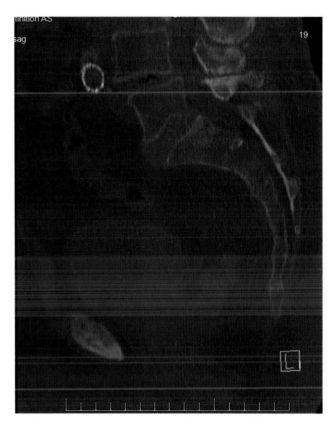

FIGURE 35–5. Sagittal MPR along the midline of the patient.

position the slice overlay perpendicular to the coronal plane. Extend the slice overlay from the iliac crest through the great trochanter (Figure 35–5).
- Use 3-dimensional shaded surface display (SSD) or volume rendering (VR).
- If there is a suspected vascular or bladder injury, then intravenous (IV) contrast may be helpful; a CT angiogram may also be performed.

Contrast Media

Usually, no contrast is used unless there is a suspected vascular or bladder injury. Retrograde filling of the bladder and CT cystography with a contrast agent may be helpful in detecting contrast extravasation, indicating bladder rupture.

Radiation Reduction Options

- Use iterative reconstruction technique to reduce radiation exposure.
- Dose modulation (tube current modulation) may be helpful in reducing radiation dose.
- Perform an AP scout only.

36

Hip

INDICATIONS

Trauma, infection, avascular necrosis, tumor, osteoporosis, and congenital and developmental abnormalities.

IMAGING APPLICATIONS

Patient/Part Positioning

Position the patient supine and headfirst in the gantry. Position the legs flat and the affected hip in the center of the table. If possible, position the pelvis into a true anteroposterior (AP) position with the feet rotated 15 to 20 degrees medially and secured together. If performing a bilateral hip exam, axial and coronal images will include both hips. Sagittal images will be performed on each hip individually.

Scan Range

Perform an AP scout from the iliac crest to the proximal femur (Figure 36–1). For axial images, align the slice overlay to be parallel to the roof of the acetabulum. Extend the axial oriented slice overlay from the anterior inferior iliac spine (approximately 3-5 cm) above the superior rim of the acetabulum to a point just below (3-5 cm) the lesser trochanter (Figure 36–2). Further, the AP scout image (Figure 36–2) shows example for bilateral hips as demonstrated in Figure 36–3A. If only performing a single hip exam (Figure 36–3B), place the slice overlay over that hip and adjust the field of view (FOV) to cover that anatomic area.

Gantry Angulation

Gantry angulation is 0 degrees.

Field of View (FOV)

The field of view is usually 12 to 25 cm.

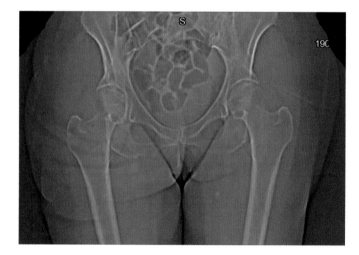

FIGURE 36–1. AP scout of pelvis for bilateral hip exam.

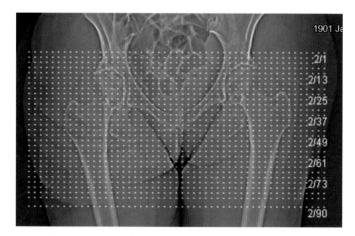

FIGURE 36–2. AP scout of the pelvis with axial slice overlay for bilateral hip exam. Note that the field of view (FOV) can be adjusted for either a single hip or bilateral hips.

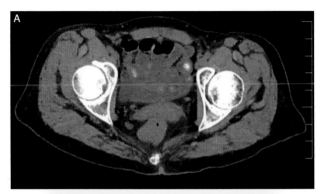

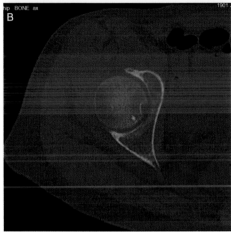

FIGURE 36–3. Axial image of bilateral hips (**A**). Axial image of right hip with a bone window setting (**B**) reconstructed from original data set.

Slice Thickness

Use a reconstructed slice thickness of 3 mm or less for better spatial resolution.

Table Movement

Craniocaudal.

Reconstruction Kernel/Algorithm

Soft tissue and bone algorithms should be used.

Window Level (WL)/Window Width (WW)

Approximate setting for:

- Soft tissue: +50 HU = WL; +350 HU = WW
- Bone window: +300 HU = WL; +1500 HU = WW

SPECIAL CONSIDERATIONS

- Multiplanar reconstruction (MPR): For coronal images, using an axial image at the level of the hip joint, align the slice overlay to be coronal to the joint and parallel to the femoral neck (Figure 36–4). Extend the slice overlay from the ischium through the pubic symphysis to cover the joint. For sagittal oblique images, use a coronal image that shows the femoral neck. Align the slice overlay to be parallel with the femoral neck and perpendicular to the

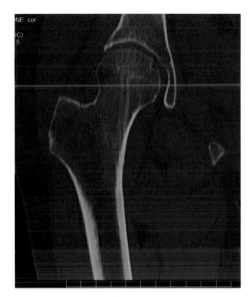

FIGURE 36–4. Coronal MPR of the right hip. Note the greater trochanter and the concave depression known as the fovea capitis. The fovea capitis serves as an attachment point for the ligament of the head of the femur (formerly known as the ligamentum teres), which holds the femur in the acetabulum. In addition, key blood vessels from the acetabulum pass along the ligamentum teres to the fovea capitis to provide blood to the head of the femur.

acetabulum (Figure 36–5). Extend the slice overlay to include the acetabulum and the greater trochanter.

- Shaded surface display (SSD) may be helpful.
- Volume rendering (VR) may be helpful.

Contrast Media

No contrast is used for bony evaluation.

Radiation Reduction Option

- Gonadal shielding positioned on the anterior surface of the female patient may be used.

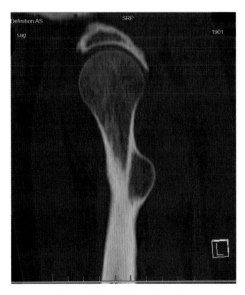

FIGURE 36–5. Sagittal MPR of the right hip. Note the space between the acetabulum and the head of the femur and the lesser trochanter.

37

Knee

INDICATIONS

Trauma and nontraumatic abnormalities, pain, soft tissue injury, follow-up from a previous injury, bone tumor, presurgery planning, and if an MRI is contraindicated.

IMAGING APPLICATIONS

Patient/Part Positioning

Position the patient supine and feetfirst in the gantry. Keep legs together and straight on the CT table. Position the affected knee so it will be in the center of the table. Adjust the patient's leg with a slight internal rotation so the femoral epicondyles are parallel with the CT table.

Scan Range

For axial images, align the slice overlay to be parallel to the tibial plateau (Figures 37–1 and 37–2). Scan from just above the patella through the tibial tuberosity and proximal tibiofibular joint.

Gantry Angulation

Gantry angulation is 0 degrees, parallel with the tibial plateau.

Field of View (FOV)

Adjust the FOV to the size of the knee. Usually, an FOV of 16 cm or smaller is acceptable. On larger individuals or in cases of swelling, a larger FOV may be needed.

Slice Thickness

Use a reconstructed slice thickness of 3 mm or less for better spatial resolution.

Table Movement

Craniocaudal.

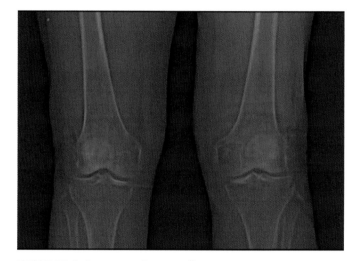

FIGURE 37–1. Anteroposterior scout of knees.

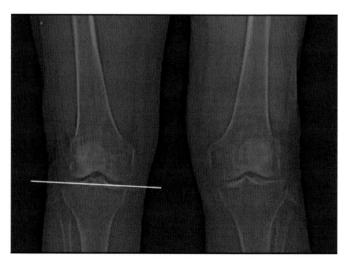

FIGURE 37–2. Anteroposterior scout of knees showing slice alignment for axial reconstructions of right knee.

Reconstruction Kernel/Algorithm

Soft tissue and bone algorithms should be used.

Window Level (WL)/Window Width (WW)

Approximate setting for:

- Soft tissue: +50 HU = WL; +350 HU = WW
- Bone window: +300 HU = WL; +1500 HU = WW

SPECIAL CONSIDERATIONS

- Multiplanar reconstruction (MPR): For coronal images, using an axial image showing the femoral condyles (Figure 37–3), align the slice overlay to be parallel with the transcondylar axis. Extend the slice overlay to cover the entire knee. See Figure 37–4, A and B. For sagittal images, using an axial image showing the femoral condyles (see Figure 37–3), align the slice overlay to be perpendicular with the transcondylar axis. Extend the slice overlay to cover the entire knee. See Figure 37–5.
- Use the metal artifact reduction algorithm to reduce metal artifact from implants or other metal objects.
- Use 3-dimensional shaded surface display (SSD) or volume rendering (VR) for preoperative planning.

Contrast Media

No contrast is used for bony evaluation.

Radiation Reduction Options

No recommendations.

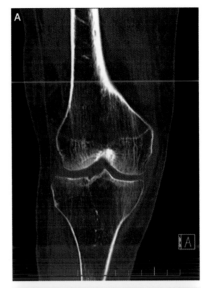
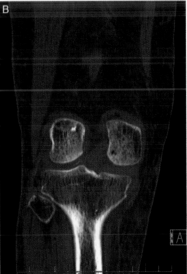

FIGURE 37–4. (**A and B**) Coronal MPR images of the knee. Image A is anterior to image B. Note the proximal tibiofibular joint in image B.

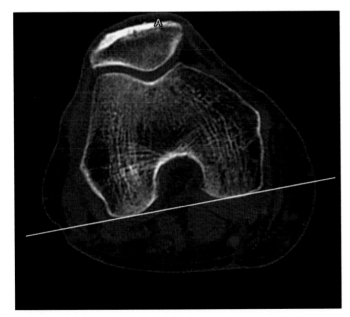

FIGURE 37–3. Axial image (bone window) showing joint space between the patella and the medial and lateral femoral condyles. Note that the line is parallel to the posterior aspect of the femoral condyles (transcondylar axis) in preparation to reconstruct coronal MPR images.

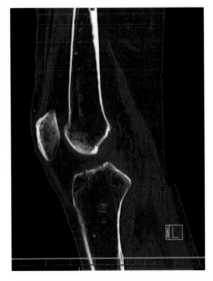

FIGURE 37–5. Sagittal MPR of the knee.

38
Ankle

INDICATIONS

Trauma and nontraumatic abnormalities, pain, soft tissue injury, follow-up from a previous injury, bone tumor, presurgery planning, and if an MRI is contraindicated.

IMAGING APPLICATIONS

Patient/Part Positioning

Position the patient supine and feet or foot of interest first into the gantry. Center the feet or foot of interest to the center of the table with the foot pointing up and immobilized to help control for motion. A relaxed position may be used if the patient is unable to flex their foot (Figure 38–1).

Scan Range

For axial images, align the slice overlay parallel to the tibiotalar (ankle) joint. Extend the slice overlay to scan from the distal tibia through the calcaneus (Figure 38–2).

Gantry Angulation

Gantry angulation is 0 degrees, parallel to the ankle tibiotalar joint.

Field of View

The field of view is small, depending on the size of the ankle (usually 10-16 cm).

Slice Thickness

Use a reconstructed slice thickness of 3 mm or less for better spatial resolution.

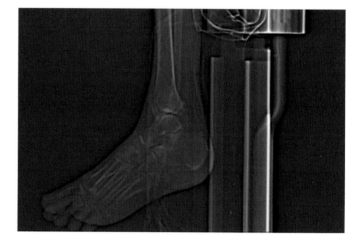

FIGURE 38–1. Lateral scout of the ankle in the relaxed position.

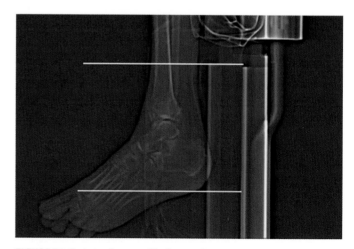

FIGURE 38–2. Lateral scout with slice overlay.

Table Movement

Craniocaudal.

Reconstruction Kernel/Algorithm

Soft tissue and high-resolution bone algorithms.

Window Level (WL)/Window Width (WW)

Approximate setting for:

- Soft tissue: +50 HU = WL; +350 HU = WW
- Bone window: +300 HU = WL; +1500 HU = WW

SPECIAL CONSIDERATIONS

- Multiplanar reconstruction (MPR): For sagittal MPR images, using an axial image (Figure 38–3) at the level of the lateral and medial malleoli and talus, align the slice overlay parallel to the inferior tibiofibular joint. Extend the slice overlay to cover the entire foot. See Figure 38–4. For coronal MPR images, using an axial image (see Figure 38–3) at the level of the lateral and medial malleoli and talus, align the slice overlay perpendicular to the inferior tibiofibular joint. Extend the slice overlay from the calcaneus through the base of the metatarsals. See Figure 38–5.
- Shaded surface display (SSD)
- Volume rendering (VR)

Contrast Media

No contrast is used for bony evaluation.

Radiation Reduction Options

No recommendations.

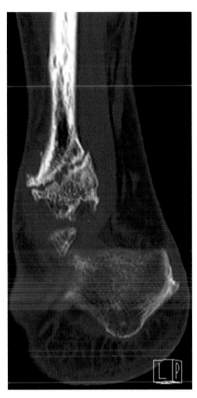

FIGURE 38–4. Sagittal MPR showing a fracture of the lateral malleolus.

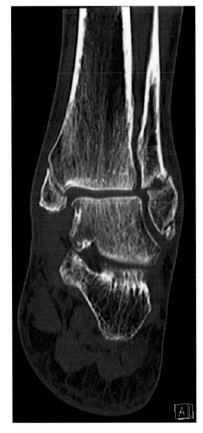

FIGURE 38–5. Coronal MPR showing fractures of the medial and lateral malleoli.

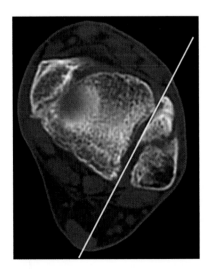

FIGURE 38–3. Axial image showing a fracture of the lateral malleolus. The line indicates the slice overlay alignment through (parallel to) the tibiofibular joint prior to reconstructing the sagittal images. The slice overlay would be extended to cover the entire ankle anatomy.

39
CT Angiography (Extremities)

INDICATIONS

Trauma and to evaluate abnormalities or injuries to the arterial system.

IMAGING APPLICATIONS

Patient/Part Positioning

Positioning depends on the extremity. For upper extremities, position the patient headfirst. For lower extremities, position the patient feetfirst. Position the patient supine. If possible, center the extremity of interest along the long axis of the table so it is in the center of the table.

Scan Range

Depends on the extremity. Include the joint nearest the area of concern.

Gantry Angulation

Gantry angulation is 0 degrees.

Field of View

Depends on the extremity. All anatomy of the extremity being imaged should be included.

Slick Thickness

Use a reconstructed slice thickness of 3 mm or less for better spatial resolution.

Table Movement

Depends on the extremity. Caudocranial for upper extremities. Craniocaudal for lower extremities.

Reconstruction Kernel/Algorithm

Soft tissue and bone algorithms should be used.

Window Level (WL)/Window Width (WW)

Approximate setting for:

- Soft tissue: +50 HU = WL; +350 HU = WW
- Bone window: +300 HU = WL; +1500 HU = WW

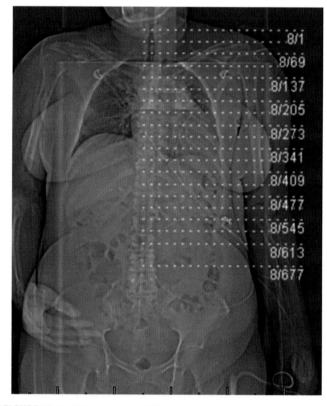

FIGURE 39–1. Anteroposterior (AP) scout with slice overlay for proximal upper extremity. Note that the scan range on this example is longer than necessary and adds additional radiation exposure to the patient. Further, it is important to note that in this example the patient's thorax and abdomen are being scanned (scanned field of view [SFOV]), the dotted lines represent the displayed FOV (DFOV). Finally, to reduce radiation dose to the patient and improve image quality, the patient's right upper extremity could have been raised over their head.

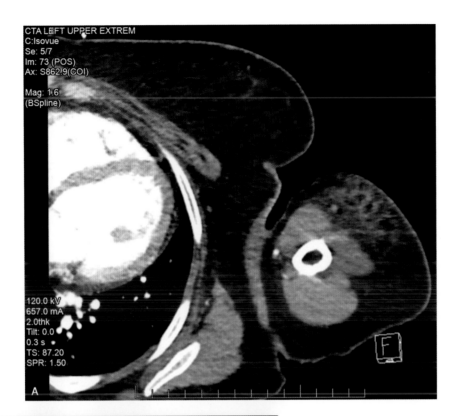

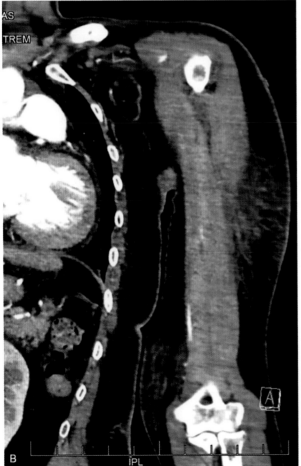

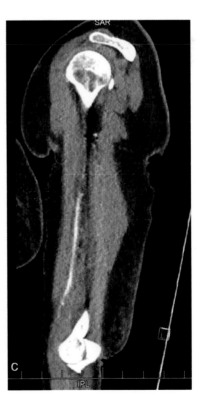

FIGURE 39–2. Axial CT angiography (CTA) of the left upper extremity (**A**), coronal image (**B**), and sagittal image (**C**).

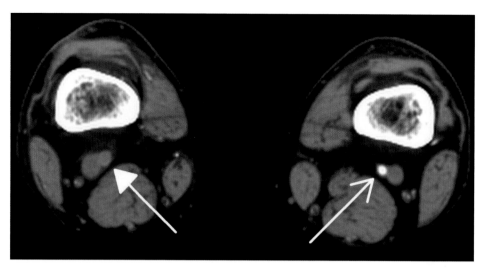

FIGURE 39–3. Axial CT angiography of the lower extremities. In comparison images, the right side shows an occlusive vessel, whereas the left side is patent. (Reprinted from Grey ML, Alinani JM. *CT & MRI Pathology: A Pocket Atlas*. McGraw-Hill; 2018, with permission from The McGraw-Hill Companies.)

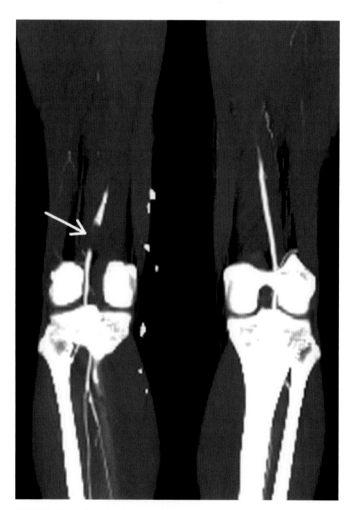

FIGURE 39–4. Same patient as in Figure 39–3. Coronal images show occlusive area on the right side. (Reprinted from Grey ML, Alinani JM. *CT and MRI Pathology: A Pocket Atlas*. McGraw-Hill; 2018, with permission from The McGraw-Hill Companies.)

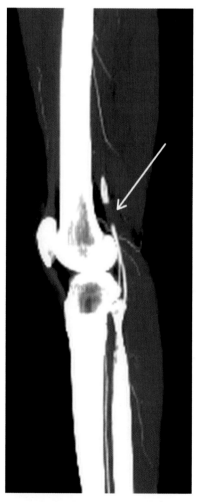

FIGURE 39–5. Same patient as in Figures 39–3 and 39–4. Sagittal image shows occlusive area. (Reprinted from Grey ML, Alinani JM. *CT and MRI Pathology: A Pocket Atlas*. McGraw-Hill; 2018, with permission from The McGraw-Hill Companies.)

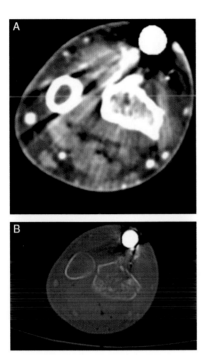

FIGURE 39-6. Left distal upper extremity with gunshot injury showing large metallic foreign body in the dorsal sift tissue over the radius; soft tissue window (**A**) and bone window (**B**).

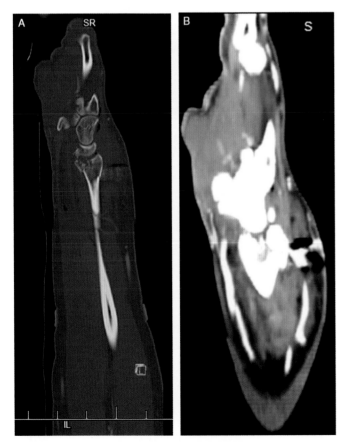

FIGURE 39-7. Same patient as in Figure 39-6. Sagittal maximum intensity projection (MIP) bone window showing comminuted fractures of the distal radius involving the articular surface and the lunate (**A**). Sagittal MIP soft tissue window (**B**) showing the radial and ulnar arteries intact and without laceration.

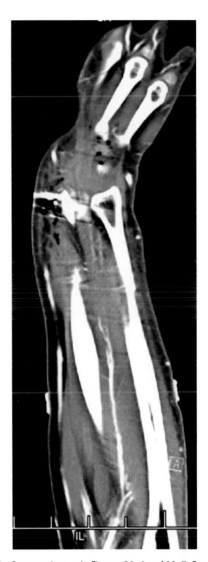

FIGURE 39-8. Same patient as in Figures 39-6 and 39-7. Coronal maximum intensity projection (MIP) soft tissue image showing intravenous contrast-filled vessel between the radius and ulna.

SPECIAL CONSIDERATIONS

- Coronal and sagittal multiplanar reconstruction
- Curved planar reconstruction
- Coronal and sagittal maximum intensity projection

Contrast Media

Intravenous (IV) contrast injection may be 4 to 5 mL/s with a chaser of normal saline. Bolus triggering region of interest (ROI) is positioned proximal to the extremity of interest.

Radiation Reduction Options

- Use iterative reconstruction technique to reduce radiation exposure.
- Dose modulation (tube current modulation) may be helpful in reducing radiation dose.

PART III

Registry Review

CT Review Questions

1. Of the following, which CT scanner is known for its "rotate-rotate" type motion?
   A. First-generation CT
   B. Third-generation CT
   C. Fourth-generation CT
   D. Ultrafast CT

2. What CT unit is slip-ring technology incorporated into?
   A. Fourth-generation CT
   B. Dynamic scanning
   C. Electron beam technology
   D. Spiral CT

3. How are the attenuation characteristics of tissues best represented?
   A. CT numbers
   B. Heat units
   C. Hounsfield units
   D. Both A and C

4. Which of the following does *not* contribute to reducing the patient dose during imaging?
   A. Automatic tube modulation
   B. Patient centering
   C. 1:1 pitch
   D. Repeating the exam

5. Which of the following has the highest CT number?
   A. Cerebrospinal fluid
   B. Brain gray matter
   C. Liver
   D. Calcified pineal gland

6. What does the SI unit gray (Gy) best define?
   A. Absorbed dose
   B. Exposure
   C. Effective dose
   D. Both A and B

7. When considering reducing radiation dose, which of the following would *not* reduce radiation dose when using CT in the "spiral" mode?
   A. Shielding
   B. Iterative reconstruction
   C. Oversampling
   D. Tube modulation

8. What effect does an increase in the number of pixels (matrix size) have on spatial resolution?
   A. Increases
   B. Decreases
   C. Remains the same
   D. Has no effect on resolution

9. What artifact will occur if a thick-slice axial data set is reconstructed into MPR images?

 A. Z-axis

 B. Ring

 C. Stair step

 D. Beam hardening

10. Of the following, which is *not* a 3-dimensional reconstruction method commonly used in CT angiography?

 A. Maximum intensity projection (MIP)

 B. Shaded surface display

 C. Volume rendering

 D. MPR

11. What CT number is water assigned?

 A. −1000

 B. −100

 C. 0

 D. +100

12. How would coronal imaging of the carpal bones be performed?

 A. Position the anatomic structure in a coronal position

 B. MPR

 C. MIP

 D. Rotate the axial images

13. What CT component is primarily responsible for the mathematical calculations involved in image reconstruction?

 A. Analog-to-digital converter

 B. Array processor

 C. Digital-to-analog converter

 D. Data acquisition system

14. What does the window level best control?

 A. Density

 B. Spatial resolution

 C. Contrast

 D. Tissue attenuation characteristics

15. When compared to diagnostic radiography, which of the following is better produced in CT images?

 A. Low contrast resolution

 B. Density

 C. Patient dose reduction

 D. Spatial resolution

16. Prior to image reconstruction, what component is used to change the signal produced by the detectors to numeric information?

 A. Central processing unit

 B. Analog-to-digital converter

 C. Array processor

 D. Digital-to-analog converter

17. Given a CT image displayed with a window level (WL) of 50 and a window width (WW) of 500, which of the following statements is correct?

 A. Pixels with values between 50 and 500 Hounsfield units (HU) appear white.

 B. Only tissues with attenuation characteristics between 50 and 500 HU are visualized.

 C. Pixels with values between −200 and +300 HU are assigned shades of gray.

 D. Only pixels with values between −1000 and 50 and between +500 and +1000 HU are visible.

18. Of the following, which CT number range would most likely be assigned to calcium-containing tissues?

 A. +700 to +1000 HU

 B. +100 to −300 HU

 C. −100 to +100 HU

 D. −1000 to −700 HU

19. What software command function measures tissue attenuation characteristics?

 A. Distance

 B. Histogram

 C. Field of view

 D. Region of interest

20. Of the following, which is *not* one of the common awareness programs initiated to reduce radiation dose?

 A. Formal Education

 B. Diagnostic Dose Levels

 C. Image Gentle

 D. As Low As Reasonably Achievable

21. When choosing a window to display a CT image, what best defines the width?

 A. Midpoint of the range of pixels

 B. Range of CT numbers (pixels) to be displayed

 C. Range of HU within the region of interest (ROI)

 D. Average CT number of the tissue of interest

22. Of the following, which technological advancement led to the development of spiral CT?

    1. Slip-ring technology
    2. Electron beam technology
    3. High-efficiency x-ray tubes

    A. 1 only
    B. 1 and 2
    C. 1 and 3
    D. 1, 2, and 3

23. Which dose-reduction technique should be used specifically when performing a CT chest, abdomen, and pelvis exam on a male adult?

    A. Tube modulation
    B. Retrospective scanning mode
    C. Shielding
    D. Phasic studies

24. What is used in conventional CT to control slice thickness?

    A. Table movement
    B. Collimation
    C. Fan beam
    D. Computer processing unit

25. What term best describes a 5-mm slice thickness with a 10-mm table movement?

    A. Gap
    B. Contiguous
    C. Overlap
    D. Simultaneous

26. What pitch ratio would a 10-mm table movement with a 5-mm collimation best represent?

    A. 1:1
    B. 1:2
    C. 1:1.5
    D. 2:1

27. Which of the following would a pitch ratio of 1:1 best represent?

    A. 5-mm table movement with 5-mm slice thickness
    B. 5-mm table movement with 10-mm slice thickness
    C. 10-mm table movement with 10-mm slice thickness
    D. Both A and C

28. What device is used to measure high contrast resolution?

    A. Water bottle phantom
    B. Low-contrast phantom
    C. Bar phantom
    D. SMPTE pattern test

29. Which is an example of a deterministic effect of radiation?

    A. Cataracts
    B. Leukemia
    C. Hereditary effects
    D. Cancer

30. In multidetector CT, what term is used to define the smallest single detector?

    A. Channel
    B. Detector
    C. Array
    D. Element

31. What does the SI unit Sievert best measure?

    A. Absorbed dose
    B. Exposure
    C. Effective dose
    D. Both A and C

32. How do metal artifacts appear on a CT image?

    A. Signal voids
    B. Streaks
    C. Herringbone pattern
    D. A single line

33. Which of the following can produce beam-hardening artifacts?

    A. When bone is penetrated
    B. When fat is penetrated
    C. When lung tissue is imaged
    D. When muscle tissue is imaged

34. Which of the following is a primary characteristic of spiral CT when compared to conventional CT?

    A. Continuous rotation of the x-ray tube
    B. High kVp
    C. High mAs
    D. Thin-slice imaging

35. Of the following characteristics, which contributes to the dissipation of heat in a CT x-ray tube?

   A. Beam collimation
   B. High kVp
   C. Increased beam filtration
   D. Large diameter of the anode

36. Which of the following does the ability to visibly discern 2 objects a small distance apart best associate with?

   A. Uniformity
   B. Linearity
   C. Signal-to-noise
   D. Spatial resolution

37. Which of the following best refers to scintillation detectors?

   A. Convert x-ray energy into light that in turn is converted into electrical energy
   B. Convert x-ray energy into electrical energy
   C. Incorporate the use of xenon gas under pressure
   D. Exhibit a quantum detection efficiency of 50% to 60%

38. Which reconstruction technique defines the process in which the brightest value in a series of voxels is selected and viewed in a 3-dimensional data set?

   A. Shaded surface display
   B. Maximum intensity projection
   C. Volume rendering
   D. Multiplanar reconstruction

39. Which reconstruction method is becoming more commonly used in CT today?

   A. Fourier transform
   B. Back-projection
   C. Iterative
   D. Filtered back-projection

40. Which of the following techniques may be helpful in reducing radiation dose when imaging the chest, abdomen, and pelvis of a young patient?

   A. Tube current modulation
   B. Reduced mAs
   C. Iterative reconstruction
   D. Both A and C

41. Which image quality factor best defines the ability of the CT scanner to freeze motion?

   A. Spatial resolution
   B. Contrast resolution
   C. Temporal resolution
   D. Freeze resolution

42. What is quantitative CT best used to demonstrate?

   A. Bone density
   B. Three-dimensional volume surface area
   C. Attenuation of the x-ray beam
   D. Blood flow

43. How can partial volume averaging artifact best be reduced?

   A. Decreasing the slice thickness
   B. Using a pitch ratio of 1:1
   C. Using intravenous (IV) contrast
   D. Decreasing the field of view

44. What term is used in conventional CT to describe the effect of missing a small lesion during patient respiration?

   A. Patient motion
   B. Slice-to-slice misregistration
   C. Interscan movement
   D. Back-projection error

45. Of the following, which is not a characteristic of spiral CT?

   A. Volumetric scanning
   B. Increased uniformity of IV contrast enhancement
   C. Reduced load on the x-ray tube
   D. MPR

46. Of the following, which is a disadvantage of CT?

   A. Image manipulation
   B. Low contrast resolution
   C. Spiral geometry
   D. Imaging areas surrounded by bone

47. Of the following data storage methods, which can store the most data/images?

   A. Magnetic disk
   B. Picture archiving and communications system
   C. Zip disk
   D. Optical laser disk

48. **What is 1 megabyte of data equal to?**

    A. 1,000,000,000,000 bytes

    B. 1,000,000,000 bytes

    C. 1,000,000 bytes

    D. 1000 bytes

49. **Which of the following is best expressed in (lp/cm)?**

    A. Noise

    B. Linearity

    C. Uniformity

    D. Spatial resolution

50. **What device is used today to measure radiation exposure in CT?**

    A. Film badge

    B. Thermoluminescence dosimetry

    C. Pencil ionization chamber

    D. Geiger counter

51. **Which of the following generations of CT scanners is characteristic for producing a ring artifact?**

    A. First-generation CT scanner

    B. Second-generation CT scanner

    C. Third-generation CT scanner

    D. Fourth-generation CT scanner

52. **When comparing the relative dose among various radiographic procedures, which most likely would produce the greatest dosage to the patient?**

    A. X-ray (abdomen)

    B. X-ray (lumbar spine)

    C. CT (head)

    D. CT (pelvis)

53. **What is the acceptance limit when performing the CT number calibration test for water?**

    A. 0

    B. ±3 HU

    C. ±5 HU

    D. ±10 HU

54. **Who is given credit for developing the first CT scanner?**

    A. Roentgen

    B. Hounsfield

    C. Cormack

    D. Oldendorf

55. **What is the primary benefit when using an iterative reconstruction technique?**

    A. Reduces scan time

    B. Reduces radiation dose

    C. Reduces the amount of contrast media needed

    D. Reduces image reconstruction time

56. **What is the purpose of an analog-to-digital converter?**

    A. Convert numerical information into signal fluctuations

    B. Suppress data for high-speed transmission

    C. Be used as an output device

    D. Convert signals into numbers

57. **Which of the following is *not* considered to be a hardware component?**

    A. Mouse

    B. Computer program

    C. Cathode ray tube

    D. Keyboard

58. **How many pixels are in a 256 by 256 matrix?**

    A. 512

    B. 65,536

    C. 131,072

    D. 262,144

59. **What type of radiation was used in Hounsfield's original experiments?**

    A. Gamma rays

    B. X-rays

    C. Hertz rays

    D. Microwave rays

60. **What is the center or midpoint of the range of CT numbers used during windowing?**

    A. Window width

    B. Window level

    C. Region of interest

    D. Density

61. **Which characteristics are best associated with fourth-generation CT scanners?**

    A. Rotate-translate motion and pencil beam geometry

    B. Rotate-translate motion with fan beam geometry

    C. Fan beam geometry and continuous rotation of the x-ray tube and detectors

    D. Fan beam geometry and complete rotation of the x-ray tube around a ring of stationary detectors

62. **What term is used to describe the ability of the CT detector to convert the x-ray photons into electrical energy?**

    A. Response time

    B. Stability

    C. Dynamic range

    D. Conversion efficiency

63. **What does the term *pitch* used in spiral CT best define?**

    A. Distance the table travels during one revolution of the x-ray tube

    B. Ratio of the distance the table travels to the slice thickness

    C. Distance between 2 consecutive slices

    D. Ratio of the scan time to the slice thickness

64. **What is the pitch ratio for a table movement of 15 mm/s and a slice thickness of 10 mm?**

    A. 0.6:1

    B. 1:1

    C. 1.5:1

    D. 15:1

65. **Of the following, which is *not* used in the computer system of a CT unit?**

    A. Detectors

    B. Input-output devices

    C. Central processing unit

    D. Array processor

66. **Which of the following is true for a WW setting of 400 and a WL setting of 0?**

    A. All structures between +200 and –200 will be white.

    B. All structures between 0 and +400 will have different shades of gray.

    C. All structures between –200 and +200 will be black.

    D. All structures between –200 and +200 will have different shades of gray.

67. **What does the term *windowing* mean?**

    A. Changing the image gray scale

    B. Changing the image contrast

    C. Changing the WW, WL, or both

    D. All the above

68. **What unit of measurement is used when calculating spatial resolution?**

    A. lp/cm

    B. lp/in

    C. lp/mm

    D. lp/m

69. **Of the following, which may cause streak artifacts in CT?**

    A. Beam hardening

    B. Metal

    C. Motion

    D. All of the above

70. **In CT, which of the following phrases best explains low contrast resolution?**

    A. Resolve small structures

    B. Separate small differences in tissue contrast

    C. Clearly seeing 2 objects separated by a small distance

    D. Discern small changes in tissue attenuation characteristics

71. **Of the following, which would best represent the CT number for bone?**

    A. –1000 HU

    B. 0 HU

    C. +100 HU

    D. +1000 HU

72. **Of the following, which best determines the slice thickness?**

    A. Filtered back-projection

    B. Collimation

    C. Beam filtration

    D. Arc of the fan beam

73. **What software function is used to measure tissue attenuation?**

    A. Distance

    B. Field of view

    C. Region of interest

    D. Maximum intensity projection

74. **Which of the following can be calculated from the full-width-at-half-maximum (FWHM) of a slice profile?**

    A. Contrast resolution

    B. Slice thickness

    C. Noise

    D. Scatter radiation

75. **Of the following materials, which is commonly used in the anode to increase its high heat storage capacity?**

    A. Molybdenum

    B. Zirconium

    C. Rhenium

    D. Graphite

76. **Which of the following section widths would cause the greatest amount of partial volume averaging?**

    A. 1 mm

    B. 3 mm

    C. 5 mm

    D. 10 mm

77. **What is the name of the reconstruction process when sagittal images are produced from a series of axial images?**

    A. Multiplanar reconstruction

    B. Volume rendering

    C. MIP

    D. Shaded surface display

78. **Of the following, which has the lowest CT number?**

    A. CSF

    B. Air

    C. White brain matter

    D. Bone

79. **What type of artifact generally appears as a dark horizontal line through the petrous ridges?**

    A. Ring artifact

    B. Beam hardening

    C. Motion artifact

    D. Metallic artifact

80. **Of the following, which helps produce a more uniform x-ray beam?**

    A. Filter

    B. Reconstruction algorithm

    C. Prepatient collimation

    D. Detector array

81. **Which of the following are benefits of thinner slice thicknesses?**

    1. Reduced partial volume averaging

    2. Improved spatial resolution

    3. Decreased scan time

    A. 1 and 2

    B. 1 and 3

    C. 2 and 3

    D. 1, 2, and 3

82. **Which of the following sets of values would best be considered normal levels for blood urea nitrogen and serum creatinine, respectively?**

    A. 14 mg/dL, 1.9 mg/dL

    B. 17 mg/dL, 0.9 mg/dL

    C. 20 mg/dL, 3.1 mg/dL

    D. 30 mg/dL, 5.2 mg/dL

83. **Which of the following must be included when obtaining informed consent for an invasive procedure?**

    1. Explanation of the examination techniques

    2. The possible risks and benefits of the examination

    3. Alternatives to the procedure

    A. 1 only

    B. 1 and 2

    C. 1 and 3

    D. 1, 2, and 3

84. **What would be the appropriate action if a patient requests the CT examination to be stopped?**

    A. Stop the procedure, remove the patient, reinstruct the patient to hold still, and then continue the study

    B. Stop the examination, remove the patient from the CT unit, and then release the patient with instructions to return to their physician

    C. Stop the procedure, comfort the patient, and contact the ordering physician and radiologist to discuss the patient's request

    D. Ignore the patient's request and finish the examination

85. **Which of the following exams would most likely require the CT gantry to be tilted during the exam?**

    A. Chest

    B. Knee

    C. Soft tissue neck

    D. Spine

86. Which of the following drug administration routes provides the most rapid absorption and action within the body?

    A. Oral

    B. Subcutaneous

    C. Intramuscular

    D. Intravenous

87. In documenting the outcome of an IV contrast study in the patient's chart, what information would not be needed?

    A. Age

    B. Gauge of the needle

    C. Flow rate

    D. Outcome of the exam

88. Which term best describes a patient having difficulty breathing?

    A. Dyslexia

    B. Dyspnea

    C. Dysphagia

    D. Dysphasia

89. Of the following types of oral contrast, which could cause peritonitis if there was a perforation of the digestive tract?

    A. Barium sulfate

    B. Gastrografin

    C. Iodinated contrast media

    D. Effervescent granules

90. What term is used to define the reduction in the number of infectious organisms without complete elimination?

    A. Immunization

    B. Sterilization

    C. Surgical asepsis

    D. Medical asepsis

91. What laboratory test uses the acronym PTT?

    A. Prothrombin time

    B. Passive tachycardia test

    C. Partial prothrombin time

    D. Partial thromboplastin time

92. Of the following medications, which may be administered to a patient experiencing a severe anaphylactoid reaction to an iodinated contrast agent?

    1. Atropine

    2. Diphenhydramine

    3. Epinephrine

    A. 1 only

    B. 1 and 2

    C. 1 and 3

    D. 1, 2, and 3

93. What is the normal range for prothrombin time (PT)?

    A. 5 to 8 seconds

    B. 11 to 13 seconds

    C. 15 to 25 seconds

    D. 21 to 35 seconds

94. Where should the suction unit used on a patient with a chest tube be placed?

    A. Below the level of the chest

    B. Above the level of the chest

    C. At the level of the chest

95. What term is used to describe the characteristics of a flowing fluid?

    A. Osmolality

    B. Viscosity

    C. Density

    D. Specific gravity

96. Why is iodine commonly used in radiopaque contrast agents?

    A. Viscosity

    B. Radiolucency

    C. High atomic number

    D. Osmolality

97. Of the following types of x-ray interactions, which produces the most scatter radiation in CT?

    A. Photoelectric

    B. Compton effect

    C. Pair production

    D. Coherent scatter

98. **Of the following body tissues/organs, which is the most radiosensitive?**

    A. Solid visceral organs

    B. Blood-forming organs

    C. Muscle tissue

    D. Central nervous system

99. **What component supplies power directly to the x-ray tube of a spiral CT scanner?**

    A. Nutating technology

    B. A/C current

    C. Slip ring

    D. Power cables

100. **How will changing the WL from −100 HU to +200 HU affect the image?**

    A. Gray to white

    B. White to black

    C. Black to white

    D. No effect

101. **How would a pulmonary embolus appear in the pulmonary artery when the patient is given IV contrast?**

    A. Hyperdense

    B. Isodense to the contrast agent

    C. Hypodense

102. **Which of the following veins is the preferred site for injecting an IV contrast agent?**

    A. Jugular

    B. Antecubital

    C. Lateral

    D. Subclavian

103. **What do the following traits best describe: posture, facial expression, eye contact, and touch?**

    A. Timing and relevance

    B. Verbal communication

    C. Intonation

    D. Nonverbal communication

104. **Which of the following is a patient history of slurred speech, brief loss of consciousness, and unilateral paralysis, which all resolve within 24 hours, most likely associated with?**

    A. TIA

    B. MI

    C. MVA

    D. CVA

105. **What is an aura an indication of?**

    A. Nosebleed

    B. TIA

    C. Vertigo

    D. Seizure

106. **Of the following tests, which provides a greater indication of renal function?**

    A. BUN

    B. Serum creatinine

    C. PTT

    D. ALT

107. **What is Benadryl used for?**

    A. Increase heart rate

    B. Decrease blood pressure

    C. Treat minor reactions to contrast agents

    D. Increase vasodilation

108. **Of the following, which would best fall in the normal range for BUN?**

    A. 3 to 5 mg/dL

    B. 5 to 10 mg/dL

    C. 6 to 24 mg/dL

    D. 15 to 30 mg/dL

109. **Of the following, which would best fall in the normal range for serum creatinine?**

    A. 0.7 to 1.3 mg/dL

    B. 1.0 to 2.0 mg/dL

    C. 1.3 to 2.5 mg/dL

    D. 1.6 to 2.3 mg/dL

110. **What is the key difference between an extravasation and an infiltration?**
    A. The amount of fluid
    B. Extravasation is the leakage of a toxic solution outside a blood vessel
    C. They are the same
    D. The severity

111. **What is the normal range for PTT?**
    A. 5 to 8 seconds
    B. 11 to 16 seconds
    C. 15 to 25 seconds
    D. 25 to 35 seconds

112. **Of the following, which would be a contraindication to using IV contrast?**
    A. Infection/abscess
    B. Tumor
    C. Multiple myeloma
    D. Trauma

113. **Loss of a large amount of blood can result in which of the following?**
    A. Hypovolemic shock
    B. Cardiogenic shock
    C. Neurogenic shock
    D. Anaphylactic shock

114. **Which lab tests should be performed prior to performing a biopsy or drainage procedure on a patient?**
    A. BUN and creatinine
    B. Creatinine and GFR
    C. PT and PTT
    D. All the above

115. **How would the severity of a patient's head injury best be recognized?**
    A. Heart rate
    B. Respiratory rate
    C. Level of vocabulary
    D. Level of consciousness

116. **Of the following characteristics, which one is most associated with veins?**
    A. No valves
    B. Thick walls
    C. Higher blood pressure
    D. Wider lumen

117. **When performing CPR, where is the heel of the hand positioned?**
    A. Level of the sternal angle
    B. Two finger widths below the xiphoid process
    C. Two finger widths above the level of the xiphoid process
    D. Mid-abdominal area

118. **What type of a drug is Benadryl classified as?**
    A. Antiemetic
    B. Antihistamine
    C. Antibiotic
    D. Analgesic

119. **Prior to starting an IV in the antecubital area, where should a tourniquet be placed?**
    A. At the injection site
    B. Just above the injection site
    C. Just below the injection site
    D. At the level of the axilla

120. **Heparin and warfarin (Coumadin) are classified as what type of drugs?**
    A. Antipsychotics
    B. Antidepressants
    C. Antianxiety agents
    D. Anticoagulants

121. **Which of the following may be used as a sedative for children?**
    A. Chloral hydrate
    B. Ipecac
    C. Adrenalin
    D. Motrin

122. **When inserting into a vein, In what direction is the bevel of an IV needle positioned?**
    A. Up
    B. Down
    C. Sideways
    D. Does not matter

123. **What is the average blood pressure for a middle-aged adult?**

    A. 100/60 mm Hg

    B. 110/90 mm Hg

    C. 120/80 mm Hg

    D. 140/90 mm Hg

124. **How does an infant's pulse compare to an adult's pulse?**

    A. Faster than an adult

    B. Slower than an adult

    C. Depends on the infant's state of alertness

    D. The same as an adult

125. **What is the average respiratory rate for an adult?**

    A. 25 to 32 breaths/min

    B. 20 to 30 breaths/min

    C. 16 to 19 breaths/min

    D. 12 to 20 breaths/min

126. **What is suggested when working with a patient with a contrast agent extravasation?**

    A. Applying a warm, moist compress to the injection site

    B. Applying a cold cloth to the injection site

    C. Documenting the extravasation in the patient's chart

    D. B and C

127. **Which of the following patients may benefit from the use of nonionic contrast agents?**

    A. Patients with histories of asthma or allergies

    B. Patients with histories of cardiac problems

    C. Patients who have had previous reactions to ionic contrast agents

    D. All the above

128. **Which of the following needles is typically used when injecting an IV contrast agent into an adult?**

    A. 16 gauge

    B. 18 gauge

    C. 20 gauge

    D. 22 gauge

129. **Which of the following best exemplifies objective data about a patient's health?**

    A. Subjective information

    B. Information from other family members

    C. Patient perception about their health

    D. Tests and procedures

130. **Which method of drug administration pertains to intramuscular, subcutaneous, and IV routes?**

    A. Topical

    B. Sublingual

    C. Transdermal

    D. Parenteral

131. **What category of contrast agent reaction involves a change in a patient's pulse, wheezing, and/or hypotension?**

    A. Mild reaction

    B. Moderate reaction

    C. Severe reaction

132. **What category of contrast agent reaction involves a patient who appears to be unresponsive, convulsing, or experiencing a cardiac arrest?**

    A. Mild reaction

    B. Moderate reaction

    C. Severe reaction

133. **What category of contrast agent reaction involves a patient complaining of dizziness, itching, or nausea and vomiting?**

    A. Mild reaction

    B. Moderate reaction

    C. Severe reaction

134. **What does the abbreviation PO mean?**

    A. Twice a day

    B. At bedtime

    C. Right eye

    D. By mouth

135. **What is the first step a technologist should take if the IV contrast agent extravasates?**

    A. Place a warm compress on the site of the infiltration

    B. Stop the IV

    C. Call for the radiologist or radiology nurse

    D. Take the patient to the emergency department

136. **What type of contrast agent is best to use in a patient with a suspected bowel perforation?**

    A. Oil based

    B. Barium

    C. Water soluble

    D. Air

137. Which of the following best applies to the term *pharmacokinetics*?

    A. Effects of a drug on the body
    B. Effects of a drug on specific tissue
    C. Movement of drugs through the body
    D. Dose rate

138. Of the following, who is given credit for inventing spiral/helical CT?

    A. Hounsfield
    B. Cormack
    C. Ledley
    D. Kalender

139. What component provides electrical power to the x-ray tube of a multirow detector CT (MDCT) scanner?

    A. Nutation ring
    B. Slip ring
    C. Detector supply
    D. Power cable

140. Who is given credit for the development of body CT?

    A. Hounsfield
    B. Cormack
    C. Ledley
    D. Kalender

141. What component is most unique in spiral CT?

    A. X-ray tube
    B. Multiple-detector system
    C. Slip ring
    D. Nutation

142. Of the following statements, which is *not* correct regarding electron beam CT (EBCT)?

    A. It performs subsecond imaging.
    B. Target rings are used in place of an anode.
    C. It was developed for brain (neurovascular) imaging.
    D. Calcium scoring is a noncontrast procedure.

143. What generation of CT scanners was first used for body scanning?

    A. First
    B. Second
    C. Third
    D. Fourth

144. Which type of CT scanners is the spiral CT design based on?

    A. Second-generation CT
    B. Third-generation CT
    C. Fourth-generation CT
    D. Electron beam CT (EBCT)

145. Which CT unit is best associated with the term *degree of detection*?

    A. Spiral CT
    B. MDCT
    C. Third-generation CT
    D. Fourth-generation CT

146. What term is used to describe voxels that have equal dimensions?

    A. Symmetrical
    B. Isotropic
    C. Grainy
    D. Smooth

147. What purpose does a gantry angulation of ±30 degrees serve?

    A. Assists with imaging applications
    B. Reduces radiation dose
    C. Decreases slice thickness
    D. Decreases scan time

148. What are collimators used for?

    A. Reduce scatter radiation
    B. Decrease scan time
    C. Improve patient positioning
    D. Image larger patients

149. Which of the following may be necessary when imaging large patients?

    A. High-voltage generator
    B. Collimation
    C. Large aperture
    D. Gantry angulation

150. **What decision should be made in a situation where a patient weighting 375 lb is scheduled for a CT scan of the brain and your patient table has a lift capacity of only 350 lb?**

    A. Refuse to scan the patient

    B. Raise the patient table to load the patient on the table

    C. Continue with the exam as ordered

    D. Discuss the situation with your supervisor and/or radiologist

151. **Which of the following methods of image reconstruction is becoming more commonly used to reduce radiation dose?**

    A. Back-projection

    B. Filtered back-projection

    C. Iterative reconstruction

    D. Fourier transformation

152. **Which of the following is the safest to use when getting an elderly patient onto the patient table?**

    A. Use a step stool

    B. Lower the patient table

    C. Lift the patient

    D. Use a wheelchair

153. **What effect does increasing (from 150 to 250 milliseconds) temporal resolution have when imaging a patient?**

    A. Decreases the motion of the structure being imaged

    B. Increases the spatial resolution of the anatomy

    C. Increases ability to see low contrast resolution

    D. Decreases slice thickness

154. **Which of the following would not be a major contributing factor in producing noise?**

    A. Number of detected x-ray photons

    B. Data acquisition system (DAS)

    C. Reconstruction kernal

    D. Patient motion

155. **What type of artifact is produced when the anatomic structure of interest in the image/slice is small/thin and the slice thickness is thick?**

    A. Partial volume averaging

    B. Beam hardening

    C. Ring

    D. Stair-step

156. **What quality control test best defines the ability to differentiate between small differences in density?**

    A. Uniformity

    B. High contrast resolution

    C. Spatial resolution

    D. Low contrast resolution

157. **What type of phantom is used to assess uniformity?**

    A. Water

    B. Catphan

    C. Low contrast resolution

    D. High contrast resolution

158. **Which type of artifact is commonly observed when imaging the internal auditory canal (IAC's) (seventh and eighth cranial nerves) with a typical brain slice thickness?**

    A. Ring

    B. Partial volume averaging

    C. Beam hardening

    D. Stair-step

159. **Which of the following is the modulation transfer function used to calculate?**

    A. Homogeneity

    B. Spatial resolution

    C. Low contrast resolution

    D. Signal-to-noise ratio

160. **What can a water phantom be used to evaluate?**

    A. Linearity

    B. Spatial resolution

    C. Low contrast resolution

    D. Signal-to-noise ratio

161. **What does the ability to differentiate between small changes in density best describe?**

    A. Signal-to-noise ratio

    B. Spatial resolution

    C. Homogeneity

    D. Low contrast resolution

162. **What does the ability to clearly see 2 objects separated by a small distance best define?**

    A. Slice thickness

    B. Spatial resolution

    C. Uniformity

    D. Low contrast resolution

163. **What is the FWHM of a slice sensitivity profile best used to calculate?**

    A. Slice thickness

    B. Signal-to-noise ratio

    C. Uniformity

    D. Linearity

164. **What effect on spatial resolution will decreasing the slice thickness have?**

    A. Increase

    B. Decrease

    C. No effect

165. **Which of the following controls partial volume averaging?**

    A. Increasing the gap between image slices

    B. Increasing the mA

    C. Decreasing the slice thickness

    D. Instructing the patient to hold their breath

166. **Which anatomic area of a CT scan of the brain would beam-hardening artifact most likely affect?**

    A. Falx cerebri

    B. Cerebellum

    C. Body of the lateral ventricle

    D. Middle cerebral arteries

167. **Where should the WL be centered when adjusting for a specific tissue?**

    A. Above the density level (Hounsfield units) of the tissue of interest

    B. Below the density level (Hounsfield units) of the tissue of interest

    C. Near the density level (Hounsfield units) of the tissue of interest

168. **What is the average HU value for a normal kidney?**

    A. 10 HU

    B. 30 HU

    C. 50 HU

    D. 70 HU

169. **How would hyperdense structures above 85 HU appear in a brain window if the WL is 35 HU and the WW is between 80 and 100 HU?**

    A. Black

    B. White

    C. Gray

170. **Do the WL and WW affect the results of the ROI values?**

    A. Yes

    B. No

    C. Depends on the reconstruction kernel

171. **How would an acute hemorrhage of the brain appear on a nonenhanced CT exam?**

    A. Hyperdense

    B. Isodense to normal blood

    C. Hypodense

    D. Isodense to CSF

172. **What happens to the image contrast as the WW widens?**

    A. Increases

    B. Decreases

    C. Depends on the WL

173. **What is the purpose of Digital Imaging and Communications in Medicine (DICOM)?**

    A. Allows communication between the technologist and the radiologist

    B. Provides a pathway for data to be sent to PACS

    C. Provides postprocessing software for additional image manipulation

    D. Connects multimodality and multivendor equipment together to facilitate data transmission

174. **What action should be taken to reduce the radiation dose caused by oversampling?**

    A. Use step-and-shoot (axial) imaging

    B. Extend the patient's arms above their head during the scout

    C. Use spiral imaging mode

    D. Reduce the mA

175. **What is the vertical movement of the patient table designed to accomplish?**

    A. Scan a large distance without repositioning the patient

    B. Lift the patient

    C. Make it easier for the patient to get on and off the table

    D. Perform biopsy procedures

176. Which of the following patients are more sensitive to radiation exposure?

A. Elderly

B. Adults

C. Teenagers

D. Children

177. When performing a CT scan of the brain, which of the following would have the greatest effect on reducing radiation dose to the orbital area?

A. Using orbital shielding

B. Activating the automatic exposure control

C. Aligning along the SOML

D. Positioning the patient supine

178. How can the sensitivity to iodine used in contrast media be increased?

A. Reduce the kVp

B. Increase the amount of contrast media

C. Increase mA

D. Decrease pitch

179. How should the size of a lesion be measured?

A. Use the region of interest tool to record the mean and standard deviation of the lesion

B. Adjust the WL and WW of the image to show only the lesion

C. Use the distance measure tool and measure the long axis and the short axis of the lesion

D. Measure the distance of the true x-axis and y-axis

180. Which of the following scanning techniques is the standard when performing a biphasic exam of the liver?

A. Arterial phase and portal venous phase

B. Noncontrast phase and arterial phase

C. Arterial phase and a delayed venous phase

D. Noncontrast phase and a delayed venous phase

181. When imaging the liver in the arterial phase, where should the bolus trigger be placed?

A. Liver

B. Inferior vena cava (IVC)

C. Portal vein

D. Aorta

182. What component should be used to best tailor IV contrast enhancement in a patient?

A. Volume rendering

B. Automatic tube modulation

C. Bolus triggering

D. Region of interest

183. Following the injection of an IV contrast agent, approximately how much time should elapse before scanning a late delayed phase exam of the liver?

A. 10 to 15 minutes

B. 3 to 5 minutes

C. 1 to 2 minutes

D. 45 seconds

184. Following the injection of an IV contrast agent, approximately how much time should elapse before scanning the liver for the arterial phase?

A. 10 to 15 seconds

B. 40 to 45 seconds

C. 55 to 65 seconds

D. 3 to 5 minutes

185. Of the following organs, which has a dual blood supply?

A. Pancreas

B. Kidney

C. Liver

D. Adrenal glands

186. What is the most common benign liver tumor?

A. Hepatocellular adenoma

B. Focal nodular hyperplasia

C. Hemangioma

D. Angiomyolipoma

187. What is the most common malignant liver tumor affecting adults?

A. Cholangiocellular carcinoma

B. Hepatocellular carcinoma

C. Hepatoblastoma

D. Lymphoma

188. What is the normal CT attenuation range for the liver?

A. 0 HU

B. 10 to 20 HU

C. 20 to 30 HU

D. 55 to 65 HU

189. **Which of the following is the most commonly injured organ as a result of blunt trauma?**

    A. Spleen

    B. Liver

    C. Pancreas

    D. Kidneys

190. **When performing a liver-only examination, what is the usual scan range?**

    A. Diaphragm to symphysis

    B. Diaphragm to portal vein

    C. Diaphragm to inferior border of the liver

    D. Mid-sternum to the adrenal glands

191. **What breathing instruction should be given when imaging the abdomen?**

    A. Suspend breathing

    B. Slow quiet breathing

    C. Full inspiration

    D. Full exhalation

192. **When performing an abdomen/pelvis exam, which type of contrast media is commonly used?**

    1. Oral

    2. IV

    3. Rectal

    A. 1 and 2

    B. 1 only

    C. 2 only

    D. 1, 2, and 3

193. **What combination of phasic exams may be used in a post–follow-up ablation for liver metastases?**

    1. Arterial phase

    2. Portal venous phase

    3. Early delayed phase

    A. 1 and 2

    B. 1 and 3

    C. 2 and 3

    D. 1, 2, and 3

194. **What combination of phasic exams may be used in a post–follow-up ablation for hepatocellular carcinoma (HCC)?**

    1. Arterial phase

    2. Portal venous phase

    3. Early delayed phase

    A. 1 and 2

    B. 2 and 3

    C. 1 and 3

    D. 1, 2, and 3

195. **What is the recommended trigger level when imaging the liver?**

    A. 10 HU

    B. 30 HU

    C. 50 HU

    D. 70 HU

196. **Which patient position is best when performing a biopsy on adrenal glands?**

    A. Prone

    B. Supine

    C. Decubitus

197. **What is the greatest risk factor when performing a lung biopsy?**

    A. Infection

    B. Acute hemorrhage

    C. Hemoptysis

    D. Pneumothorax

198. **What does intense pain and tenderness at McBurney's point most likely indicate?**

    A. Appendicitis

    B. Kidney stone

    C. Pneumonia

    D. Hiatal hernia

199. **Which of the following would benefit greatly from a high-resolution CT exam of the chest?**

    A. Pneumonia

    B. Aortic dissection

    C. Emphysema

    D. Pulmonary emboli

200. Which of the following is *not* a midline structure in the brain?

   A. Falx cerebri

   B. Tentorium cerebelli

   C. Septum pellucidum

   D. Basilar artery

201. In Figure III–1, what anatomic structure is represented by the number 1?

   A. Pons

   B. Cerebellar tonsil

   C. Medulla oblongata

   D. Cerebellar vermis

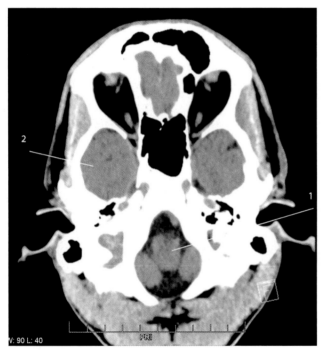

FIGURE III–1

202. In Figure III–1, what does the area labeled 2 best represent?

   A. Parietal lobe

   B. Middle fossa

   C. Sphenoid sinus

   D. Temporal lobe

203. In Figure III–2, what does the hypodense area 1 best represent?

   A. Lateral sulcus

   B. Middle cerebral artery

   C. Lateral ventricle

   D. Longitudinal fissure

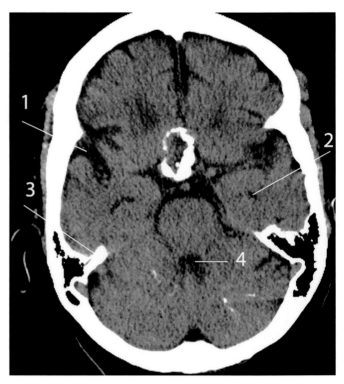

FIGURE III–2

204. In Figure III–2, what does the hypodense area 2 best represent?

   A. Confluence of sinuses

   B. Cystic lesion

   C. Quadrigeminal cistern

   D. Temporal horn

205. In Figure III–2, what does the hyperdense structure 3 best represent?

   A. Petrous ridge of the temporal bone

   B. Sphenoid wing

   C. Occipital bone

   D. Mastoid

206. In Figure III–2, what does the hypodense area 4 best represent?

   A. Quadrigeminal cistern

   B. Cerebral aqueduct

   C. Basilar artery

   D. Fourth ventricle

207. In Figure III–3, what function are line A and line B performing?

A. Distance measurement

B. Midline shift measurement

C. Measuring the distance across the brain

D. Region of interest calculation

210. In Figure III–4, what does the hypodense area 1 best represent?

A. Anterior horn of the lateral ventricle

B. Body of the lateral ventricle

C. Trigone of the lateral ventricle

D. Posterior horn of the lateral ventricle

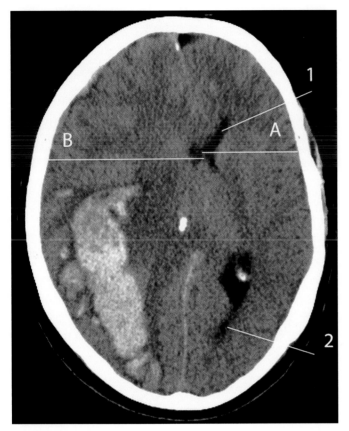

FIGURE III–3

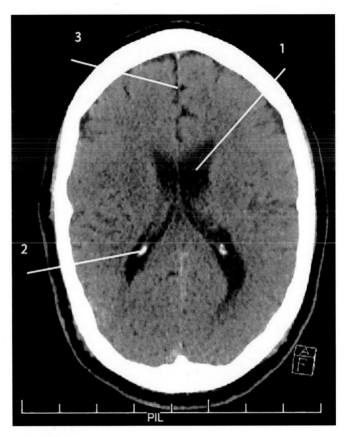

FIGURE III–4

208. In Figure III–3, what does the hypodense area 1 best represent?

A. Air

B. Third ventricle

C. Frontal horn

D. Trigone of the lateral ventricle

209. In Figure III–3, what does the hypodense area 2 best represent?

A. Posterior horn of the lateral ventricle

B. Trigone of the lateral ventricle

C. Fourth ventricle

D. Lateral ventricle

211. In Figure III–4, what does 2 best represent?

A. Choroid plexus

B. Third ventricle

C. Fourth ventricle

D. CSF

212. In Figure III–4, what is structure 3, which separates the left hemisphere from the right hemisphere?

A. Longitudinal fissure

B. Septum pellucidum

C. Third ventricle

D. Falx cerebri

213. **In Figure III–5, what part of the ventricular system is posterior to the pons?**

    A. First ventricle

    B. Second ventricle

    C. Third ventricle

    D. Fourth ventricle

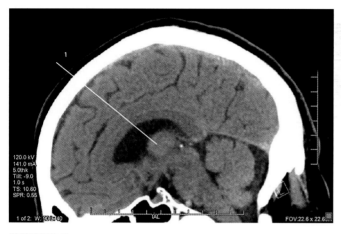

FIGURE III–5

214. **In Figure III–5, what is the name of the anatomic structure that separates the occipital lobes of the brain from the cerebellum?**

    A. Straight sinus

    B. Tentorium cerebelli

    C. Falx cerebri

    D. Meninges

215. **In Figure III–5, what neurologic structure does 1 best represent?**

    A. Caudate nucleus

    B. Optic nerve

    C. Interthalamic adhesion

    D. Pituitary gland

216. **In Figure III–6, what lobe of the brain does 1 best represent?**

    A. Frontal

    B. Parietal

    C. Temporal

    D. Occipital

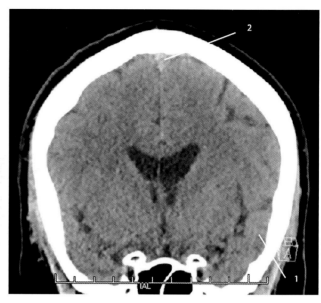

FIGURE III–6

217. **In Figure III–6, what vascular structure does 2 best represent?**

    A. Basilar artery

    B. Jugular vein

    C. Middle cerebral artery

    D. Superior sagittal sinus

218. **In Figure III–7, what image reconstruction technique was used to reconstruct this image?**

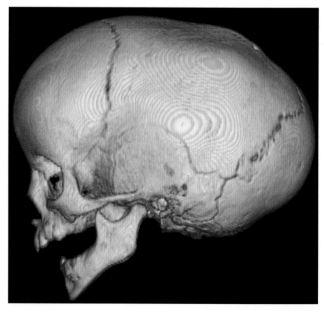

FIGURE III–7

    A. MPR

    B. Shaded surface display

    C. MIP

    D. Filtered back-projection

219. In Figure III–8, what does 1 best represent?

    A. Superior rectus muscle

    B. Medial rectus muscle

    C. Inferior rectus muscle

    D. Lateral rectus muscle

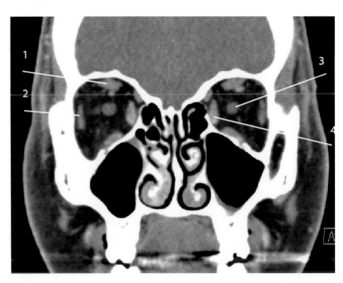

FIGURE III–9

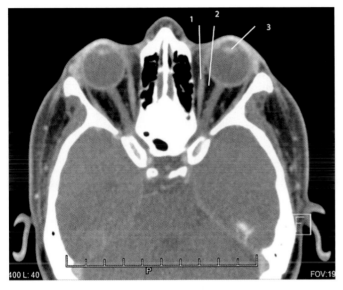

FIGURE III–8

220. In Figure III–8, what does 2 best represent?

    A. Air

    B. Cartilage

    C. Tendon

    D. Fat

221. In Figure III–8, what does 3 best represent?

    A. Lens

    B. Globe

    C. Vitreous humor

    D. Retina

222. In Figure III–9, what does 1 best represent?

    A. Superior rectus muscle

    B. Optic nerve

    C. Medial rectus muscle

    D. Lateral rectus muscle

223. In Figure III–9, what does 2 best represent?

    A. Medial rectus muscle

    B. Optic nerve

    C. Lateral rectus muscle

    D. Inferior rectus muscle

224. In Figure III–9, what does 3 best represent?

    A. Medial rectus muscle

    B. Superior rectus muscle

    C. Lateral rectus muscle

    D. Optic nerve

225. In Figure III–9, what does 4 best represent?

    A. Optic nerve

    B. Medial rectus muscle

    C. Inferior rectus muscle

    D. Lateral rectus muscle

226. In Figure III–10, what does 1 best represent?

    A. Sphenoid bone

    B. Mastoid air cells

    C. Temporal bone

    D. Occipital bone

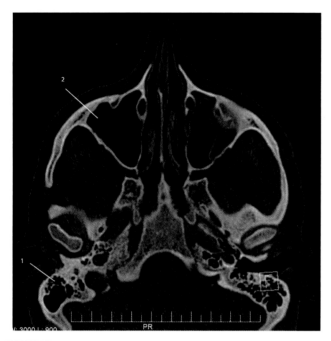

FIGURE III-10

227. In Figure III-10, what does 2 best represent?

A. Ethmoid sinus

B. Maxillary sinus

C. Sphenoid sinus

D. Frontal sinus

228. In Figure III-11, what does the hypodense 1 area best represent?

A. Oropharynx

B. Nasopharynx

C. Laryngopharynx

D. Trachea

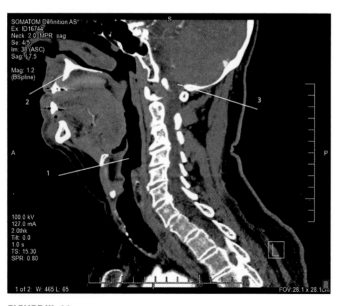

FIGURE III-11

229. In Figure III-11, what does the structure 2 best represent?

A. Nasal septum

B. Clivus

C. Sphenoid bone

D. Maxilla

230. In Figure III-11, what does the opening 3 best represent?

A. Foramen magnum

B. Jugular foramen

C. Carotid canal

D. Vertebral canal

231. In Figure III-12, what does the structure 1 best represent?

A. Brachiocephalic vein

B. Common carotid artery

C. Jugular vein

D. Subclavian artery

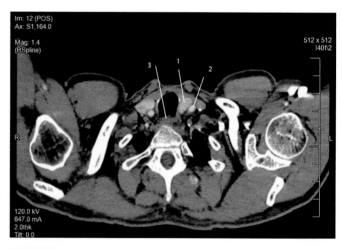

FIGURE III-12

232. In Figure III-12, what does the structure 2 best represent?

A. Brachiocephalic vein

B. Common carotid artery

C. Brachiocephalic artery

D. Jugular vein

233. **In Figure III–12, what does the structure 3 best represent?**

    A. Esophagus

    B. Common carotid artery

    C. Subclavian artery

    D. Brachiocephalic artery

234. **In Figure III–13, what does the structure 1 best represent?**

    A. Ascending portion of the aortic arch

    B. Brachiocephalic vein

    C. Subclavian artery

    D. Pulmonary trunk

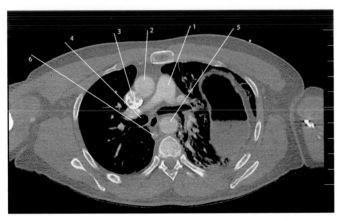

FIGURE III–13

235. **In Figure III–13, what does the structure 2 best represent?**

    A. Descending portion of the aortic arch

    B. Brachiocephalic vein

    C. Pulmonary trunk

    D. Ascending portion of the aortic arch

236. **In Figure III–13, what does the structure 3 best represent?**

    A. Pulmonary trunk

    B. Right atrium

    C. Superior vena cava

    D. Main bronchus

237. **In Figure III–13, what does the structure 4 best represent?**

    A. Right main bronchus

    B. Esophagus

    C. Trachea

    D. Carina

238. **In Figure III–13, what does the structure 5 best represent?**

    A. Inferior vena cava

    B. Descending portion of the aortic arch

    C. Descending aorta

    D. Pulmonary trunk

239. **In Figure III–13, what does the structure 6 best represent?**

    A. Vertebral artery

    B. Descending portion of the aortic arch

    C. Esophagus

    D. Azygos vein

240. **In Figure III–13, what does the structure in Question 239 drain into?**

    A. Right atrium

    B. Pulmonary artery

    C. Superior vena cava

    D. Inferior vena cava

241. **In Figure III–14, what does the structure 1 best represent?**

    A. Inferior mesenteric artery

    B. Ureter

    C. Superior mesenteric artery

    D. Celiac trunk

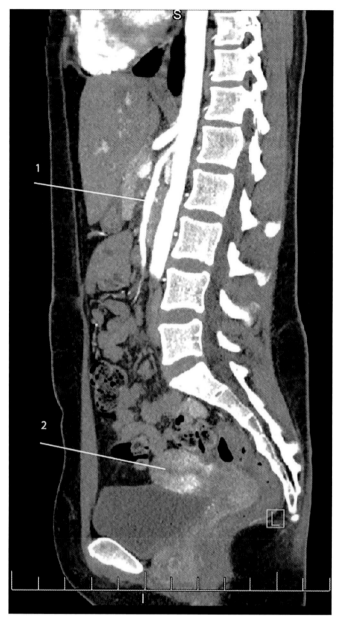

FIGURE III–14

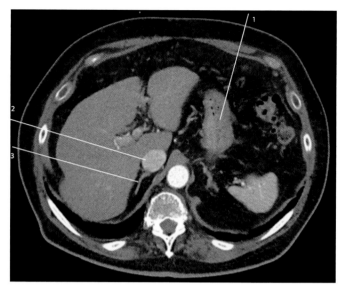

FIGURE III–15

242. **In Figure III–14, what does the structure 2 best represent?**

    A. Sigmoid colon
    B. Prostate gland
    C. Seminal vescicle
    D. Uterus

243. **In Figure III–15, what structure does 1 best represent?**

    A. Stomach
    B. Pancreas
    C. Spleen
    D. Small bowel

244. **In Figure III–15, what does the structure 2 best represent?**

    A. Descending aorta
    B. Portal vein
    C. Inferior vena cava
    D. Kidney

245. **In Figure III–15, what does the structure 3 best represent?**

    A. Kidney
    B. Adrenal gland
    C. Renal vein
    D. Splenic vein

246. **In Figure III–16, what does the structure 1 best represent?**

    A. Superior mesenteric artery
    B. Splenic artery
    C. Celiac artery
    D. Inferior mesenteric artery

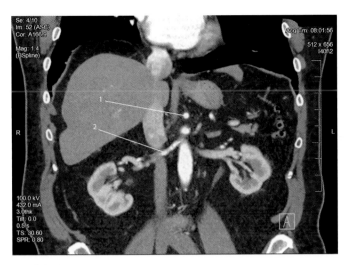

FIGURE III–16

247. **In Figure III–16, what does the structure 2 best represent?**

   A. Renal artery

   B. Splenic artery

   C. Ureter

   D. Small bowel

248. **In Figure III–17, what does the structure 1 best represent?**

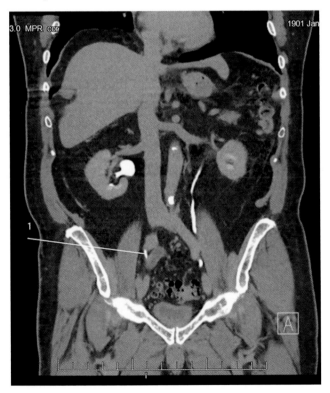

FIGURE III–17

   A. Common iliac artery

   B. External iliac artery

   C. Common iliac vein

   D. Ureter

249. **In Figure III–18, what does the structure 1 best represent?**

   A. Common iliac artery

   B. External iliac artery

   C. Femoral vein

   D. Common iliac vein

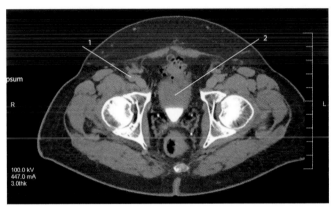

FIGURE III–18

250. **In Figure III–18, what does the structure 2 best represent?**

   A. Urinary bladder

   B. Prostate

   C. Uterus

   D. Rectum

CT Answer Explanations

1. **B** – The first 4 generations of computerized axial tomography (CAT), commonly referred to as conventional CT today, are defined according to the specific characteristics that differed between each generation. Each generation of CT scanners or CT units is characterized by key advancements in the evolution of CT, specifically how the x-ray tube and detectors move. Rotate-rotate motion describes the motion of the x-ray tube and the detector array.

2. **D** – What could be defined as sixth-generation CT is spiral CT. The x-ray tube in spiral CT can move in a circular fashion around the patient on a track continuously. This was a major technologic advancement that opened the way for new imaging applications. The terms *spiral* and *helical* can be used when describing current CT.

3. **D** – These terms may be used interchangeably when describing tissue attenuation; however, Hounsfield Units (Hus) are also used when describing "windowing" an image.

4. **D** – Repeating the exam implies that there was a mistake or error. Repeat exams due to an error or mistake will result in an increase in the radiation dose and secondly may also require additional intravenous (IV) contrast agent needing to be administered to the patient. If the exam is being performed again at a later time or date, then it is most likely referred to as a follow-up or delayed exam.

5. **D** – Calcified structures will be denser. When using the region of interest (ROI), the HUs or CT number would be higher than for other tissue.

6. **A** – The gray (Gy) is the International System of Units (SI units) unit of measure used to measure the amount of energy absorbed; the conventional system uses the rad. For example, if a patient had been administered a treatment plan (years ago) in radiation therapy for 4000 rads, that would be equal (today) to 40 Gy using the SI system (where 100 rads equals 1 Gy).

7. **C** – Spiral CT functioning in the spiral mode will "oversample" the patient's anatomy. In doing so, x-ray exposure to anatomy outside the intended scan range occurs.

8. **A** – As the number of pixels increases, the size of each pixel decreases, thus increasing the spatial resolution. For example, a 1024 × 1024 matrix has better spatial resolution than a 512 × 512 matrix.

9. **C** – The thicker the slice thickness of the original data set, the more pronounced is the stair-step artifact. The thinner the slice thickness of the original data set, the less obvious is the artifact.

10. **D** – Multiplanar reconstruction (MPR) is a 2-dimensional technique. All of the other techniques are 3-dimensional.

11. **C** – Water is used to calibrate CT scanners. The HU value of 0 is set for water. This allows for all scanners to be the same when referring to ROI.

12. **B** – The MPR technique allows the original data set to be re-reconstructed in any orthogonal plane orientation.

13. **B** – The array processor has long been known as a high-speed calculator or processor designed to rapidly perform image reconstruction computations.

14. **A** – The window level (WL) and window width (WW) are used to adjust the density and contrast of an image, respectively.

15. **A** – CT is better able to detect the sensitivity of tissues with different tissue densities than diagnostic radiography.

16. **B** – An analog-to-digital converter is used to convert analog (sign wave) data into digital data prior to image reconstruction.

17. **C** – Structures less than –200 HUs will appear black (hypodense), whereas structures greater than +300 HUs will appear bright (hyperdense). Structures between –250 and +300 HUs will appear as a shade of gray.

18. **A** – The denser the material, the higher is the HU value.

19. **D** – The ROI is used to measure the density of the pixels within the area of interest. The ROI is useful in determining a differential diagnosis of the area under investigation. The greater the number of pixels within the region, the better is the accuracy. Using a single pixel is not recommended due to statistical fluctuations. Positioning the ROI accurately within the area of interest is important for better results. Note: Do not confuse the ROI with the concept of windowing; they are different.

20. **A** – Various radiation dose reduction methods have been developed; however, formal education in CT and registration in CT have not been acknowledged as standards.

21. **B** – The WW defines which pixels will be displayed in the gray scale. Pixels below the WW will be seen as black (hypodense), whereas pixels above the WW will be seen as white (hyperdense).

22. **C** – Conventional CT, or computerized axial tomography (CAT) as it was known prior to slip-ring technology, was hindered by x-ray tube heat and interscan time delay issues. The advancements made in the x-ray tube design and ability of tube cooling along with the continuous rotation of the x-ray tube were significant advancements. The name CAT was changed to CT to better reflect the impact of these technologic advancements. Increased computer speed for faster image reconstruction and soft advancements also contributed greatly.

23. **A** – Tube modulation with the patient's arms positioned above their head prior to the scout image allows for the fluctuation of the mAs throughout the exam.

24. **B** – Prepatient and postpatient detector collimators are used to adjust slice thickness.

25. **A** – A slice thickness (SLT) of 5 mm and a table movement of 10 mm leave a gap of 5 mm between slices. This historic method of imaging was rarely used; however, when it was used, it primarily was used to cover more anatomy due to limited x-ray tube heating capacity.

26. **D** – In 1999, the International Electrotechnical Commission (IEC) introduced a definition for pitch as: pitch equals distance of table travel per tube rotation divided by total collimation. Thus, 10-mm table travel divided by 5-mm collimation equals 2, or a pitch ratio of 2:1.

27. **D** – A pitch ratio of 1:1 indicates equal table travel and tube rotation. While both A and C are correct, another question might ask: Which option would produce an image with better spatial resolution? The correct answer would be A.

28. **C** – The bar phantom is used to measure high contrast resolution. Each grouping of bars (line pairs) can be visually assessed by observing how well each group of bars is able to be seen. Spatial resolution can be simply evaluated by assessing the smallest grouping and clearly seeing 3 of 5 pairs of lines as separate and distinct.

29. **A** – Severity of an effect increases with the dose. Radiation dose and tissue sensitivity are important issues when performing CT. Factors such as patient/part positioning, scan range (oversampling or overranging), and mode of scan (axial vs helical) are important to consider for each patient.

30. **D** – As an example, a 16 multirow detector system with 912 channels would have 14,592 individual elements.

31. **C** – Effective dose relates to exposure to risk. See deterministic effects of radiation.

32. **B** – Use of a metal artifact reduction (MAR) program can help reduce this type of artifact.

33. **A** – The denser the tissue, the greater is the tissue attenuation that leads to beam-hardening artifact.

34. **A** – The main advantage of spiral CT is the slip-ring technology, which provides for continuous rotation of the x-ray tube.

35. **D** – In addition to other factors, the larger and thicker anode helps displace heat better.

36. **D** – Spatial resolution defines how well small structures can be clearly seen.

37. **A** – Scintillation detectors (or more commonly known as solid-state detectors) are only used in current CT units. Gas ionization detectors are no longer used.

38. **B** – Maximum intensity projection (MIP) is a commonly used technique in CT angiography postprocessing.

39. **C** – Due to radiation dose concerns, iterative reconstruction techniques have been implemented by all manufacturers.

40. **A** – Using tube current modulation will allow the fluctuation of the mAs based off the attenuation of the anatomy generated during the scout image. Iterative reconstruction uses a computer algorithm to help overcome the noise associated with filtered back-projection type of image reconstruction without increasing the radiation dose. Iterative reconstruction techniques allow the amount of radiation dose previously used with filtered back-projection reconstruction technique to be reduced. Question: For medicolegal purposes, how are either of these radiation dose reduction techniques documented on the image?

41. **C** – Temporal resolution is measured in milliseconds and applied to cardiac imaging. The faster the x-ray tube rotation time, the better is the ability to freeze cardiac motion. A 100-millisecond temporal resolution CT system would be better than a 200-millisecond temporal resolution CT system.

42. **A** – Quantitative CT is used to measure the bone density for osteoporosis.

43. **A** – Small lesions may be difficult to see if the voxel (slice thickness) is greater than the size of the lesion. This

happens as a result of the averaging of the data within the thickness of the slice of tissue and when the contribution of data representing the lesion is not significant enough to affect the outcome. It represents only a partial amount of the slice thickness but not enough.

44. **B** – In conventional CT, a single slice acquisition was acquired per tube rotation. The x-ray tube would then have to rewind the power cable and the table advance to begin a new slice. The time between slices was called the interscan time delay. The patient would be given breathing instructions regarding when to breathe and when to hold their breath throughout the entire exam. Small lesions located near the diaphragm, either above or below, could be missed because of different inhalation breaths (thus the term *slice-to-slice misregistration*).

45. **C** – With the development of slip-ring technology, continuous x-ray tube rotation provided the ability for new advancements in imaging options. One of the biggest advancements was angiographic imaging. Longer imaging times meant greater workload on the x-ray tubes. X-ray tubes today are much better at withstanding higher tube heat and much better at tube cooling than ever before.

46. **D** – Beam hardening artifacts occur when imaging near areas with bone. This artifact reduces the quality of the image.

47. **B** – Picture archiving and communication systems (PACS) have an unlimited amount of data storage capability as compared to other historical methods.

48. **C** – Image storage historically required calculating the amount of data needed for each image (eg, 256 × 256 matrix or 512 × 512 matrix). An approximate number of slices per exam was then calculated along with the number of patients imaged per week in order to purchase enough storage material, such as magnetic tape and zip disks. PACS provide an endless amount of storage.

49. **D** – Spatial resolution indicates how many pairs of lines can be clearly seen in 1 cm (lp/cm). The more pairs of lines that can be seen, the higher (greater) is the spatial resolution.

50. **C** – The pencil ionization chamber is an instrument used to record radiation exposure. It is placed in a phantom and to measure the dose of a given technique.

51. **C** – The rotate-rotate type of scanners produces ring artifact. The x-ray tube and the detectors would rotate around the patient. If one of the detectors malfunctioned, there would be a noticeable dark ring seen as a result of the loss of data for that single slice.

52. **D** –. The thickness and amount of bony anatomy would most likely require more radiation dosage to adequately produce diagnostic images as compared to the other options in the question. Other procedures such as

multiphasic exams, angiography exams, and exams combining the chest, abdomen, and pelvis would be greater in radiation dose. Thus, using tube modulation, iterative reconstruction, and performing the exam correctly the first time are beneficial in reducing dose.

53. **B** – This quality control (QC) test evaluates the ROI function on a water bottle phantom. The ROI of the phantom should be within ±3 HUs of 0 HU. This helps to assure that the ROI function is accurate when being used.

54. **B** – Dr. Godfrey Hounsfield's research resulted in the development of the first clinically useful CT scanner. Dr. Allan Cormack, a professor and mathematician, developed the solutions to the mathematical problems for image reconstruction in CT. Both Hounsfield and Cormack were awarded the Nobel Prize in Medicine and Physiology in 1979 for their contributions in developing CT.

55. **B** – Filtered back-projection was the technique used for image reconstruction and was used for many years; however, as computer speed increased, the iterative reconstruction (IR) technique became more feasible. Manufacturers now offer the iterative reconstruction technique as a method to help reduce radiation dose to the patient.

56. **D** – See earlier answer explanation for Question 16.

57. **B** – A computer program is software.

58. **B** – The number of pixels in a matrix is an indication of the spatial resolution of the monitor. The greater the number of pixels, the better is the spatial resolution.

59. **A** – The initial research used a gamma source; however, it took a very long time to scan an object. The gamma source was replaced with an x-ray tube.

60. **B** – The WL is the midpoint, whereas the WW is the range of CT numbers.

61. **D** – The various generations of CT scanners have been grouped according to the characteristics of the x-ray tube and detectors. In conventional CT, specific generations of CT scanners were described. Answer A is first generation. Answer B is second generation. Answer C is a slip-ring (spiral/helical) CT scanner since the x-ray tube demonstrates continuous rotation.

62. **D** – Response time is the speed of a detector to detect an x-ray and recover and be able to repeat and detect another exposure. Stability refers to the steadiness of the detector during an exposure without the need for frequent calibrations. Dynamic range is the ability of the detector to measure the precision of the largest to the smallest x-ray signal.

63. **A** – Pitch is the distance of table travel to one rotation of the x-ray tube. For example, if the table moved 10 mm in one tube rotation and the slice thickness is 10 mm, then this would be an example of a 1:1 pitch ratio.

64. **C** – Calculate: 15 mm ÷ 10 mm = 1.5:1 pitch ratio.

65. **A** – The detectors are located within the CT gantry.

66. **D** – See earlier answer explanation for Question 17 and compare. Structures with CT numbers below –200 HU will be black (hypodense), and structures with CT numbers above +200 HU will be white (hyperdense).

67. **D** – Windowing involves adjusting the WW and WL to change the gray scale and the image contrast so the anatomic tissue is more clearly seen.

68. **A** – Using lp/mm is too small of a scale of measurement.

69. **D** – The appearance of streak artifacts is important to note; however, knowing what caused the streak artifact is more important.

70. **D** – Differences in tissue attenuation result in tissues with different densities. These differences in density determine image contrast. Small changes in tissue attenuation would be associated with low contrast (increased number of the shades of gray). Answer B is more associated with quality control (QC) testing.

71. **D** – See earlier answer explanation for Question 18 and compare. The higher the HU number, the more radiodense is the structure.

72. **B** – Of the choices given, the collimation system's main function is to set the slice/section thickness. It also assists with reducing scatter radiation.

73. **C** – The ROI is helpful in providing information about the tissue. The CT number (+/– HU) represented in the ROI is an indicator of the type of tissue.

74. **B** – The "real" slice thickness can be calculated using the full-width-at-half-maximum (FWHM) sensitivity profile.

75. **D** – Graphite has a much higher heat storage capacity than tungsten.

76. **D** – As the slice thickness increases, the chance of missing small lesions also increases. As a side note, review the concept of FWHM with contiguous imaging.

77. **A** – The MPR technique allows images to be re-reconstructed in any orientation (orthogonal).

78. **B** – Air would have a negative ROI value on the Hounsfield scale.

79. **B** – This artifact may appear in the region of the brainstem during a CT exam of the brain. As a suggestion, there are ways to reduce this artifact, for example, using thinner slice thickness, repositioning the patient's head so the orbitomeatal line (OML) is vertical and the gantry is at a zero tilt, or starting imaging below the external occipital protuberance and continuing through the petrous ridges. These modifications should be approved by the radiologist prior to performing.

80. **A** – A filter is used to help provide a uniform beam of x-ray before interacting with the patient.

81. **A** – Imaging a patient with thin slice thickness would most likely increase the scan time due to the range of scanning.

82. **B** – The normal blood urea nitrogen (BUN) range for a patient is 6 to 24 mg/dL. The normal range for serum creatinine is 0.7 to 1.3 mg/dL.

83. **D** – Explaining alternatives to the procedure can only be performed by a qualified physician. This means that the technologist or a nurse cannot perform the function of obtaining an informed consent from the patient.

84. **C** – Contacting the radiologist and ordering physician is advised. In the event that neither of them can be contacted, contacting your supervisor regarding the situation would be the next option. In addition, document the request and any further information regarding this situation in the patient chart.

85. **D** – The CT gantry is tilted when imaging parallel through the intervertebral joint space, especially the cervical and lumbar spine.

86. **D** – Medications and fluids administered directly into the bloodstream are immediately available for use by the body.

87. **A** – Because the biographical information is already in the patient's chart, the patient's age would not need to be documented. The total volume of the contrast agent, saline flush, and any particular information that may be helpful, including injection site, should be documented.

88. **B** – Dyspnea is the medical term used to define difficult or labored breathing. What do the other terms define?

89. **A** – Barium sulfate is not soluble in water. If it is suspected that the patient may have a perforation of the bowel or the patient has a known perforation of the bowel, it is recommended that barium not be used.

90. **D** – Medical asepsis is known as the clean technique. Surgical asepsis, also known as sterile technique, is the complete killing of microorganisms.

91. **D** – Partial thromboplastin time (PTT) is used to measure clotting time in a blood sample. Normal range is 60 to 70 seconds. A value of more than 70 seconds signifies a chance of spontaneous bleeding.

92. **D** – In the event of any reaction to iodinated contrast media, the radiologist should be contacted immediately. In addition, it is recommended to follow the radiology department policy when it is suspected that a patient has a contrast reaction.

93. **B** – In patients not taking blood-thinning medications, the normal range for prothrombin time (PT) is 11 to 13.5 seconds. The higher the PT time, the longer it takes for the blood to clot. The PT and PTT may be required prior to biopsy procedures in CT.

94. **A** – Caution is necessary when handling a patient with a chest tube so as not to compromise the integrity of the tube and equipment. Keep the suction below the level of the chest for proper drainage.

95. **B** – The viscosity of IV contrast media may be thick and difficult to inject into a patient's vein. Usually, contrast warmers are used to help reduce the viscosity so the contrast media flows easier into the patient.

96. **C** – The high atomic number attenuates the x-ray beam.

97. **B** – Compton effect or Compton scatter is the main cause of scatter radiation. It occurs due to the interaction of the x-ray or gamma photon with free electrons (unattached to atoms) or loosely bound valence shell (outer shell) electrons.

98. **B** – In the group of options provided for this question, blood-forming tissues and organs would be the most sensitive. What types of cancers are commonly seen in populations exposed to radioactive material?

99. **C** – Third-generation CT scanners were successfully modified with the development of slip-ring technology to provide continuous rotation of the x-ray tube. All spiral/helical CT scanners today are based off the third-generation concept. Nutating technology was tried with fourth-generation CT scanners to provide continuous x-ray tube rotation but failed.

100. **B** – The WL adjusts the density of the image.

101. **C** – The pulmonary embolism (PE) (clot) would appear darker (hypodense) than the bright (hyperdense) IV contrast media.

102. **B** – The antecubital area of the elbow is the more common location to inject an IV contrast agent. The veins in that location can more easily accommodate a large-gauge needle than the veins in the back of the hand. A larger-gauge needle will allow a higher injection rate without causing discomfort to the patient.

103. **D** – Nonverbal communication is helpful to the technologist in determining the status of the patient.

104. **A** – This patient history indicates a transient ischemic attack (TIA). These may be referred to as mini strokes.

105. **D** – An aura is a condition that often occurs before a migraine or seizure.

106. **B** – Of the listed tests, creatinine provides a better indicator of overall kidney function. Although the blood urea nitrogen (BUN) is also an indicator of kidney function, its value may change more rapidly due to fluid intake. Before the estimated glomerular filtration rate was available, technologists would rely more commonly on the patient's creatinine level.

107. **C** – A physician may use Benadryl to treat minor reactions to contrast media.

108. **C** – This is considered to be the normal range; however, the range may vary depending on other factors.

109. **A** – The normal range is 0.7 to 1.3 mg/dL.

110. **B** – If a toxic solution leaks out of a vein, this is referred to as an extravasation. IV contrast agent are considered to be toxic to tissue outside the vein. Chemotherapy agents are toxic, and if they leak during treatment, it is referred to as an extravasation. Leak of a nontoxic solution, such normal saline, is referred to as an infiltration.

111. **D** – This blood test provides information about the patient's blood clotting ability. In a patient not taking any prescribed blood thinner, their PTT should be approximately 25 to 35 seconds. For a patient on a blood thinner, their clotting time may be 2.5 times longer.

112. **C** – Multiple myeloma is a contraindication to using iodine-based contrast media. This is due to a possible risk for postcontrast acute kidney injury. Some studies suggest that modern nonionic iodine-based contrast media can safely be administered to patients with multiple myeloma who have normal renal function. Verify with your radiologist.

See *European Radiology* 2018;28:683-691.

113. **A** – Hypovolemic shock may occur if the volume of blood is too small. Cardiogenic shock may result due to heart problems. Neurogenic shock may result from damage to the nervous system. Finally, anaphylactic shock may result from an allergic reaction.

114. **C** – See earlier answer explanations for Question 93 and 111.

115. **D** – The Glasgow Coma Scale provides a practical method for assessment of impairment of level of consciousness in response to defined stimuli. It is based on a patient's (1) eye opening, (2) verbal response, and (3) motor response.

116. **D** – Veins have valves, thin walls, and lower blood pressure as compared to arteries.

117. **C** – Place the heel of the hand on the sternum just above the xiphoid process.

118. **B** – An antihistamine is a drug used primarily to treat allergic disorders.

119. **B** – The tourniquet is placed above the site, tying it tight enough to slow the venous blood flow and loose enough to not impede arterial blood flow.

120. **D** – Anticoagulants are drugs that inhibit clotting of the blood.

121. **A** – Chloral hydrate is commonly used as a sedative for children. It is useful when a child needs to be very still for 20 to 60 minutes.

122. **A** – The bevel, or slanted part at the tip of the needle, is to be positioned facing up prior to inserting it into the patient. This guards against plugging the bore of the needle with skin tissue and then possibly injecting it into the patient's vein.

123. **C** – A systolic/diastolic blood pressure of less than 120/80 mm Hg is normal. Hypotension or low blood pressure occurs if the blood pressure is below 95/60 mm Hg.

124. **A** – The younger a child, the faster is their pulse rate. As the child gets older, their pulse rate begins to slow down.

125. **D** – Silent, effortless, and regular respiratory rates of 12 to 20 breaths per minute are normal for an adult.

126. **D** – Apply a cold cloth, elevate the extremity, contact the radiologist, and document the specifics of the incident in the patient's chart. Failure to document the details of the venipuncture procedure and extravasation in the patient's chart could result in medicolegal consequences.

127. **D** – With the approval of the radiologist, nonionic contrast agents may be beneficial when imaging patients with various health conditions and prior history of reaction to ionic contrast media. Currently, nonionic contrast agents are the standard iodinated agent.

128. **B** – For most CT exams, an 18-gauge needle is sufficient for an adult patient. A 20-gauge needle will most likely be too small when used with a power injector.

129. **D** – Tests and outcomes of procedures on the patient provide objective information. All the other options are subjective.

130. **D** – Topical drugs are applied to the skin. Sublingual drugs are given under the tongue.

131. **B** – Patients showing moderate reactions require immediate treatment.

132. **C** – Severe reactions are life threatening.

133. **A** – Mild reactions require observation to ensure they do not progress. The radiologist does need to be contacted to evaluate the patient.

134. **D** – The abbreviation PO means by mouth. For example, NPO means nothing by mouth.

135. **B** – Stop any additional contrast media from entering the patient.

136. **C** – A water-soluble contrast agent such as Gastrografin or an iodinated contrast agent may be helpful.

137. **C** – For example, iodinated IV contrast media do not dissociate and are excreted through the kidneys by glomerular filtration. This is usually performed over a certain period of time depending on the contrast agent and patient's renal function.

138. **D** – Dr. Kalender, a medical physicist who worked for Siemens Medical Solutions in Erlangen, Germany, is given credit for inventing spiral/helical CT.

139. **B** – The slip ring replaced the need for the power cable to connect directly to the x-ray tube.

140. **C** – The first-generation CT scanner was a "head-only" design. Dr. Ledley worked to extend the ability of CT scanning to the body. His CT scanner became known as a second-generation scanner.

141. **C** – Suppling electrical power to the slip ring, instead of the traditional power cable connection to the tube, reduced scan time and advanced medical imaging.

142. **C** - This is an historical question. The electron beam CT (EBCT) scanner or ultrafast CT scanner was specifically designed to image the heart. This was due to the increased health issues associated with heart disease. Electron beam BCT was the first attempt at what is now known as cardiac imaging in CT.

143. **B** – This is an historical question. Dr. Ledley is given credit for advancing CT to be able to image the body.

144. **B** – The movement of the x-ray tube and detector array was called "rotate-rotate" for the third-generation CT units. This is because both the x-ray tube and the detector array rotated around the patient. The fourth-generation scanners were called "rotate-stationary" or "rotate only." Manufacturers of CT scanners at the time were producing either third-generation or fourth-generation scanners.

145. **D** – This is an historical question. *Degree of detection* was a term used specifically with fourth-generation CT scanners. The detectors in a fourth-generation scanner do not move, in contrast to the third-generation CT units or spiral CT today. Instead, the detectors are fixed and attached inside the gantry area. As detector technology advanced, they became smaller. Initially, there were 360 detectors, one for each degree of the circle surrounding the gantry. As the technology continued to advance and the detectors became smaller, more detectors were added to each degree. So, if a CT unit has a full degree of detection, it has 360 detectors. If the unit has half a degree of detection, there are 720 detectors. Quarter degree of detection indicates 1440 detectors. As detector size decreases and the number of detectors increases, spatial resolution increases accordingly.

146. **B** – Isotropic imaging provides superior spatial resolution. The x-, y-, and z-axes of the voxel are equal in size.

147. **A** – Angling the CT gantry to image parallel through an anatomic area such as the vertebral joints provides superior spatial resolution. As an interesting note, CT scanners that cannot angle their gantry were primarily designed for body imaging, such as imaging the chest, abdomen, and pelvis, and the vascular studies associated with them.

148. **A** – Collimators are also useful in reducing scatter radiation. This improves the quality of the image.

149. **C** – Design of CT scanners was advanced to assist with imaging bariatric patients. Larger patients required larger apertures and greater table lift capacities.

150. **D** – Patient table weight capacities need to be taken into consideration to safely image a patient when the weight of the patient exceeds the table lift capacity. Otherwise, there is risk of the table breaking or being damaged, which can result in unnecessary risks to the patient and medicolegal risks for the providers involved.

151. **C** – With advanced computer technology, computer speed, the ability to perform reconstruction calculations faster, allows iterative reconstruction techniques to be used, which allows reduction of radiation dose to the patient.

152. **B** – Knowledge of the patient table can be helpful in providing a safe imaging environment for the patient. Knowledge of how it operates, its safe lift capacity, and extent of tabletop travel distance is important in everyday imaging. Lowering the table to a height approximately level to the back of the patient's knee will safely help in loading and unloading a patient.

153. **A** – Increasing temporal resolution allows for motion-free cardiac imaging.

154. **D** – Patient motion may appear as streaks and/or a blurring of the detail of the image.

155. **A** – The smaller the structure, the less the attenuation contributes to the overall reconstruction of the image. Thus, lesser contribution results in reduced ability to visualize the structure.

156. **D** – The Catphan phantom is used to evaluate low contrast detectability.

157. **A** – Using a water bottle phantom, use the ROI to measure the CT numbers of an image of the water bottle at the 3, 6, 9, and 12 o'clock and center positions. Record the mean (HU) number and the standard deviation for each position. The values should be 0 HU with a standard deviation of ±2 (−2 to +2 would be the acceptable range).

158. **B** – Because the seventh and eighth cranial nerves are very small and the typical thickness of a slice for a brain is 8 mm, a partial volume averaging artifact most likely will result in not clearly being able to see those cranial nerves. Thin-section images help to reduce partial voluming.

159. **B** – The modulation transfer function can be used to compare the performance of different CT systems' spatial resolution.

160. **D** – A water bottle phantom can be used to calculate the signal-to-noise ratio. Using the ROI, measure the mean signal within the water bottle phantom. Then measure the mean and standard deviation outside the phantom (background). Subtract the mean of the background from the mean of the signal producing area of the water bottle and then divide by the standard deviation of the background.

161. **D** – The ability to detect small differences in density helps in detecting lesions. Contrast agents may also be used to help detect lesions.

162. **B** – Spatial resolution defines the ability to see small structures. Measuring spatial resolution can be accomplished using the modulation transfer function or by measuring the lp/cm.

163. **A** – For example, if you were scanning in the axial mode using a 10-mm slice thickness (SLT), what would the real slice thickness be? It is not 10 mm. It will be less than 10 mm. If you are performing contagious imaging (eg, 10-mm slice thickness with a 10-mm table movement), you could possibly miss a small lesion.

164. **A** – Decreasing slice thickness also decreases partial voluming, which allows smaller structures to be better seen.

165. **C** – Decreasing slice thickness also decreases partial voluming.

166. **B** – Dense bone surrounding the brainstem and cerebellum would mostly be affected.

167. **C** – The mean (average) density level of the WL should be set as close as possible to the density level of the tissue to be examined.

168. **B** – The mean density HU of the kidney is 30 ± 10 HUs (20-40 HU).

169. **B** – All structures hyperdense to 85 HU would appear white.

170. **B** – Adjusting the WL and WW does not affect the results of the ROI.

171. **A** – Acute bleeds will be hyperdense (bright).

172. **B** – Widening the WW (eg, increasing from 100 to 400 HU) increases the number of shades of gray. Narrowing the WW (eg, from 1000 to 100 HU) would decrease the number of shades of gray.

173. **D** – Digital Imaging and Communications in Medicine (DICOM) regulations required manufacturers to design equipment so that medical imaging equipment purchased from a variety of manufacturers would be able to communicate with each other.

174. **A** – Oversampling is inherent when using the spiral/helical mode of scanning.

175. **C** – The vertical movement of the patient table is designed to assist patients in getting on and off the table. A patient would have less difficulty getting on or off the table if it can be lowered to a safe level. If a patient's weight is greater than the lifting capacity of the table, it is suggested that the patient table not be raised to its highest level and then the patient transferred over onto the patient table. This practice is dangerous and could result in the patient falling. The technologist should know the table lift capacity of the CT unit they are using. See earlier answer explanations for Questions 150 and 152.

176. D – The younger the patient being imaged, the more radiosensitive they are. In addition, the younger patient has several more years of life expectancy and may experience deterministic effects of radiation dose.

177. C – Although orbital shielding is helpful, aligning the gantry to be parallel to the supraorbitomeatal line (SOML) and avoiding the orbit provide the greatest protection from radiation exposure. See Chapter 5. If the anatomy of the eye is present on the image, the radiosensitive lens of the eyes has been exposed to radiation. The protocol for the orbits is different than that for the brain.

178. A – Lowering the kVp increases the CT numbers of the contrast-enhanced structures, thus improving the signal-to-noise ratio and potentially reducing the radiation dose.

179. C – Select an image that shows the lesion at its largest size, and then using the distance measuring tool, measure the distance along the long axis and the short axis of the lesion. In addition, use the ROI to access the "mean" of the lesion. Make sure there are several pixels within the ROI for a more accurate assessment.

180. A – Biphasic liver exams include an arterial phase and a portal phase. For triphasic exams, a nonenhanced phase is performed prior to the arterial and portal phases.

181. D – Place the bolus tracking ROI in the aorta. Shortly after this is triggered by the arrival of the IV contrast agent, the arterial phase of the exam will be acquired.

182. C – Bolus tracking, also referred to as bolus trigging, is used to monitor the IV contrast agent prior to entering the anatomic area of interest.

183. A – While an early delayed phase is 3 to 5 minutes, the late delayed phase is 10 to 15 minutes following the IV contrast injection.

184. A – Depending on the flow rate, this would be rather a short time following the beginning of the IV contrast injection. The arterial phase of scanning should begin 5 to 10 seconds after the enhancement in the bolus triggering ROI exceeds 50 HU above the baseline.

185. C – The liver has a dual blood supply, the hepatic arteries and the portal system.

186. C – Hepatic hemangiomas are the most common benign liver tumor and usually found incidentally during radiologic examination.

187. B – Hepatocellular carcinoma (HCC) is the most common primary cancer of the liver. In children, it is the second most common cancer after hepatoblastoma.

188. D – The CT attenuation for normal liver parenchyma is between 55 and 65 HU.

189. A – The liver is the second most commonly injured organ as a result of blunt trauma.

190. C – For a liver-only examination, the scan range would be from the diaphragm through to the inferior border of the liver.

191. C – Full inspiration should be performed when imaging the abdomen.

192. A – Rectally administered contrast is rarely performed.

193. C – Arterial and portal phases may be used for hypervascular lesions (HCC).

194. A – See earlier answer explanation for Question 193.

195. C – The recommended trigger level is 50 HU above the baseline.

196. B – Prone position provides the best access to the adrenal glands.

197. D – Following the removal of the needle, a follow-up scan/slice is taken at the level of the biopsy to document postbiopsy status.

198. A – McBurney's point is a landmark that is found along a straight line extending from the umbilicus to the anterior superior iliac spine (ASIS). The point is located about two-thirds the distance from the umbilicus.

199. C – Thin-section (1-2 mm) high-resolution CT (HRCT) of the lung parenchyma is usually performed with a 1- to 2-cm gap.

200. B – The tentorium cerebelli, also referred to as the "tent," separates the cerebrum above from the cerebellum below. Vascular structures of interest such as the superior sagittal sinus and the inferior sagittal sinus meet at the internal occipital protuberance and then divide to become the transverse sinuses. The falx and septum pellucidum can be used to measure midline shift.

201. C – Medulla oblongata is the distal portion of the brainstem. The foramen magnum is visible. Lateral to the medulla oblongata are the cerebellar tonsils.

202. B – Middle fossa or temporal fossa. This bony area surrounds the temporal lobe of the brain.

203. A – Lateral sulcus or Sylvian fissure separates the frontal lobe from the temporal lobe.

204. D – Temporal horn or inferior horn of the left lateral ventricle. The horn can be referred to by either name. To communicate clearly and completely, say the entire name; for example, temporal horn of the left lateral ventricle. The doctors will be impressed!

205. A – Petrous ridge of the temporal bone.

206. D – Fourth ventricle. The fourth ventricle is located posterior to the pons. The quadrigeminal cistern is superior to the fourth ventricle. The cerebral artery is anterior to the pons.

207. B – Measuring the shift of the midline is important for neurologic evaluation. Measure from a midline structure, in this case, the septum pellucidum, where the greatest shift is occurring to the internal table of the skull on one side. Record the distance in millimeters, and then repeat on the opposite side. Subtract the difference to report the midline shift.

208. **C** – Frontal horn or anterior horn of the left lateral ventricle. Each horn can be referred to by either name.

209. **A** – Posterior horn or occipital of the left lateral ventricle. Each horn can be referred to by either name. The posterior horn is the extension posteriorly from the trigone or atrium of the lateral ventricle.

210. **B** – The body of the lateral ventricle. From the body of the lateral ventricle extending anteriorly is the frontal or anterior horn. Extending posteriorly is the trigone or atrium and then the posterior horn or occipital horn. Inferiorly is the temporal horn or inferior horn. Extensive knowledge of the ventricular system of the brain was required for technologists prior to CT due to a procedure known as pneumoencephalography. Knowledge of the ventricular system of the brain is still important in CT as well as MRI.

211. **A** – The choroid plexus produces cerebrospinal fluid. Sometimes, they calcify. These are calcified choroid plexuses, an incidental finding and seen bilaterally. All 4 ventricles have a choroid plexus. The largest accumulation is found in the trigone area of the lateral ventricles.

212. **D** – The falx cerebri is the structure that separates the hemispheres of the brain. The space that the falx is in is called the longitudinal fissure. Also of interest is the superior sagittal sinus, which runs along the same course and provides venous drainage.

213. **D** – The fourth ventricle is posterior to the pons. Although the third and fourth ventricles are well known, the terms *first ventricle* and *second ventricle* are more historic and date back to initial studies of brain imaging with a technique known as pneumoencephalography. The left lateral ventricle was called the first ventricle, and the right lateral ventricle was referred to as the second ventricle. Recall that, in English, reading is from top to bottom (superior to inferior) and left to right.

214. **B** – Much like the falx cerebri, the tentorium cerebelli supports the brain.

215. **C** – The interthalamic adhesion, also known as the massa intermedia, connects the 2 lobes of the thalamus together. The massa intermedia passes through the third ventricle.

216. **C** – The Sylvian fissures bilaterally help in identifying the temporal lobes of the cerebrum.

217. **D** – The superior sagittal sinus drains venous blood posteriorly to connect with the confluence of sinuses. From the confluence of sinuses, blood flows into the left and right lateral sinuses, also known as transverse sinuses, eventually draining into the jugular veins. See earlier answer explanation for Question 212.

218. **B** – Shaded surface display is commonly used for 3-dimensional bone imaging.

219. **B** – The 4 larger muscles controlling eye movement are listed as possible answers.

220. **D** – Fat tissue, specifically retro-orbital fat. If using the ROI to access the HUs of this hypodense area, it would be approximal –90 HU to –15 HU. Air, another hypodense-appearing area, would be much lower when using the ROI to access.

221. **A** – In this CT exam of the orbits, note the difference in the applications as compared to a brain protocol. Also worth noting is the lack of orbital shielding.

222. **A** – In this coronal plane, use the concept of a clock to help identify the 4 larger rectus muscles. Example 12 o'clock (superior), 3 o'clock (medial or lateral depending on left or right eye), 6 o'clock (inferior), and 9 o'clock (medial or lateral depending on left or right eye). The optic nerve is found in the center position unless there is a space-occupying lesion or trauma. See Figure III–8 to compare. Note the metal streak artifact from dental fillings.

223. **C** – See earlier answer explanation for Question 222.

224. **D** – See earlier answer explanation for Question 222.

225. **B** – See earlier answer explanation for Question 222.

226. **B** – The mastoid air cells are within the temporal bone; however, the pointer is pointing to the hypodense air pockets.

227. **B** – Maxillary sinus. The left maxillary sinus is partially filled with air. The right side appears to be filled with air.

228. **C** – The pharynx is divided into 3 specific areas. In descending order, the nasopharynx is posterior to the nasal cavity, the oropharynx is posterior to the oral cavity, and the laryngopharynx is located posterior to the larynx. The trachea would be inferior to the laryngopharynx.

229. **D** – The hard palate of the maxilla is hyperdense and forms approximately two-thirds of the roof of the mouth. The soft palate is posterior to the hard palate. The clivus is inferior to the sphenoid sinus.

230. **A** – The foramen magnum allows the brainstem, specifically the medulla oblongata, to connect with the spinal cord and pass from the cerebrum into the spinal canal.

231. **C** – Jugular vein.

232. **B** – Common carotid artery.

233. **A** – Esophagus.

234. **D** – Pulmonary trunk.

235. **D** – Ascending portion of the aortic arch.

236. **C** – Superior vena cava.

237. **A** – Right main bronchus.

238. **B** – Descending portion of the aortic arch.

239. **D** – Azygos vein.

240. **C** – The azygos vein drains into the superior vena cava.

241. **C** – The superior mesenteric artery (SMA) is the second anterior branch off the descending aorta after passing through the aortic hiatus. The celiac trunk just above the SMA is the first anterior branch.

242. **D** – Uterus.

243. **A** – Stomach.

244. **C** – Inferior vena cava.

245. **B** – Adrenal gland.

246. **C** – Celiac artery.

247. **A** – Renal artery.

248. **D** – Ureter.

249. **B** – External iliac artery.

250. **A** – Urinary bladder.

Index

Note: Page numbers followed by *f* indicate figures; and page numbers followed by *t* indicate tables.